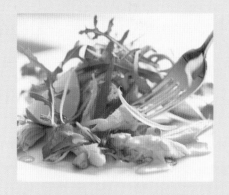

# STRONG BONES
## FOR
# LIFE

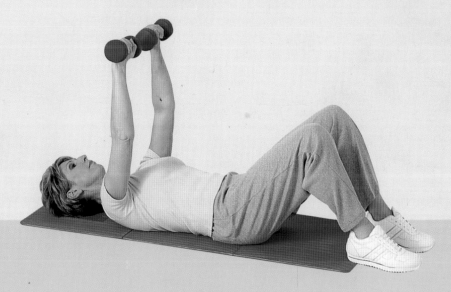

CARROLL & BROWN PUBLISHERS LIMITED

JOAN BASSEY PHD
& SUSIE DINAN

FIONA HUNTER
& EMMA-LEE GOW

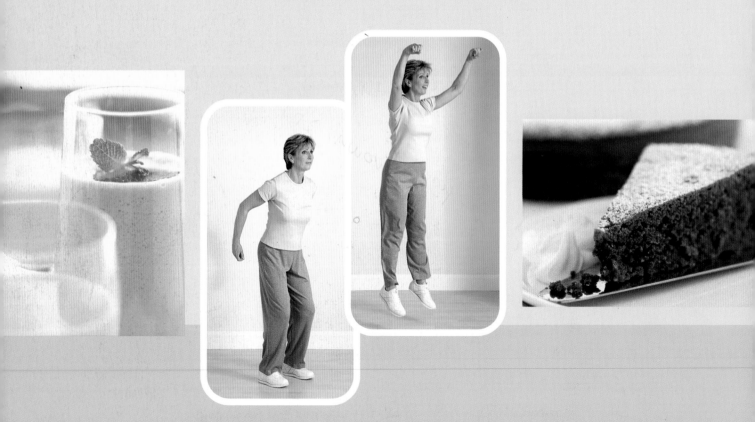

# STRONG BONES
## FOR
# LIFE

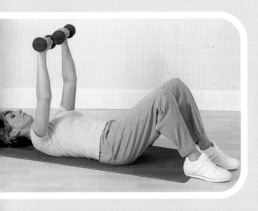

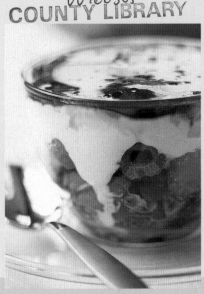

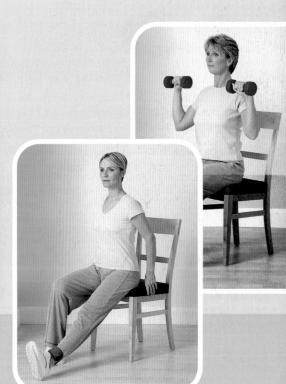

CARROLL & BROWN PUBLISHERS LIMITED

This edition first published in 2004 in the United Kingdom by:

Carroll & Brown Publishers Limited
20 Lonsdale Road
Queen's Park
London NW6 6RD

A CIP catalogue record for this book is available
from the British Library
ISBN 1-903258-95-2

Compiled from Exercise for Strong Bones and
Great Healthy Food for Strong Bones

The information in this book reflects, to the best of the authors' abilities, current scientific thinking on exercise training for reducing the risk of osteoporotic fracture in healthy women. While the recommendations are appropriate in most cases, and safe if followed as prescribed, they are not intended to replace medical advice. Neither the authors nor the publishers shall be liable or responsible for any loss, injury, or damage allegedly arising from any information or suggestion in this book.

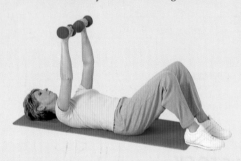

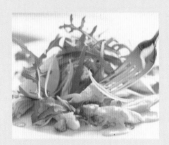

**Exercise for Strong Bones**

First published in 2001 in the United Kingdom by:
Carroll & Brown Publishers Limited

Text copyright © E. Joan Bassey and Susie Dinan 2001
Illustrations and compilation copyright © Carroll & Brown
Publishers Limited 2001

A CIP catalogue record for this book is available from
the British Library
ISBN 1-903258-38-3

The information in this book reflects, to the best of the authors' abilities, current scientific thinking on exercise training for reducing the risk of osteoporotic fracture in healthy women. While the recommendations are appropriate in most cases, and safe if followed as prescribed, they are not intended to replace medical advice. Neither the authors nor the publishers shall be liable or responsible for any loss, injury, or damage allegedly arising from any information or suggestion in this book.

**Great Healthy Food for Strong Bones**

First published in 2002 in the United Kingdom by:
Carroll & Brown Publishers Limited

**Consultant for National Osteoporosis Society** Dr Sue New

Copyright © 2002
Carroll & Brown Limited

A CIP catalogue record for this book is available from
the British Library
ISBN 1-903258-32-4

# Contents

Foreword by Linda Edwards,
Director of the National
Osteoporosis Society 6

## EXERCISE FOR STRONG BONES

What is osteoporosis? 8
Understanding your bones 9
How bone changes with age 10
Are you at risk? 11
The weak spots 13
Prevention & treatment 14
Reducing your risk 15

### GOOD PRACTICE 16
Look after your back 18
Strengthen your pelvic
   floor muscles 19

### GETTING STARTED 20

## WARMING UP 24

Walk, side-step & march 26
Shoulder & ankle mobilisers 28
Side & twist: spine
   mobilisers 30
Calf & thigh stretches 32
Side & chest stretches 34
Hamstring & tricep stretches 36

## HOME EXERCISES 38

Flamingo swing 40
Tandem stand & walks 42
Toe walks 44
Back lift 46
Flying back lift 48
Leg lift 50

Side leg lift 52
Thigh squeeze 54
Leg press 56
Leg curl 58
Straight leg lift 60
Thigh lift 62
Wrist curl 64
Arm curl 66
Arm press 68
Shoulder press 70
Chest press 72
All-fours 74
Wrist press, twist & pull 76
Abdominal lift 78
Flexibility stretches 80

## ACTIVITIES FOR LIFE 82

Walking 83
Stair climbing 84
Aquarobics & Tai Chi Ch'uan 85
Walk–jog 86
Weight-training 88
Jumping 90
Classes & Dancing 92
Running 93

Health questionnaire 94
Health problems and exercise 95
Physical activity checklist 96
Tailor your own programme 97

## GREAT HEALTHY FOOD

### FOOD FOR STRONG BONES 98

### CHAPTER 1 104
Start the Day 105

### CHAPTER 2 114
Soups & Appetizers 115

### CHAPTER 3 126
Light Snacks & Lunches 127

### CHAPTER 4 140
Main Courses 141

### CHAPTER 5 184
On the Side 185

### CHAPTER 6 194
Puddings & Treats 195

### CHAPTER 7 206
Home Bakes 207

## NUTRITIONAL ANALYSIS 218

## INDEX 222

Useful addresses 224
References 224

# Foreword

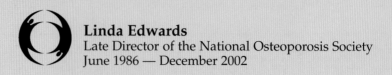

**Linda Edwards**
Late Director of the National Osteoporosis Society
June 1986 — December 2002

This book is designed to help healthy women adopt a lifestyle that will optimize bone strength and so reduce their risk of developing osteoporosis, or 'brittle bones'. Its emphasis is specifically on activities that promote bone strength and reduce the risk of fracture, and strong nutritional advice that offers further essential protection.

The exercises included in the first section are not intended to help you lose weight (that might not be a good idea for your bones anyway) but they will improve your muscle strength and give you a more streamlined look. They should make you feel more confident because your increased strength will make many physical demands and activities easier.

Dr Joan Bassey and Susie Dinan have been advising the National Osteoporosis Society (NOS) on the role of exercise in bone health since the late 1980s. Both Joan and Susie were key to the publication of two NOS publications that gave advice to those wanting to exercise to help prevent and treat osteoporosis. These booklets, used in conjunction with NOS publications offering information on diet, treatments and other aspects of osteoporosis, are essential reading for men and women concerned about their bone health. This book takes the reader further into the role of exercise and will give much needed expert guidance on developing your own bone-friendly exercise routine. The NOS is indebted to Joan and Susie for their dedicated support of the NOS and our continuing campaign to improve the prevention and treatment of osteoporosis.

The second section gives essential advice on nutrition and bone health. With over 120 recipes, all containing bone-friendly ingredients, and many low in fat, eating for strong bones will become both easy and highly pleasurable.

## THE NATIONAL OSTEOPOROSIS SOCIETY

The NOS is the UK's authoritative voice on osteoporosis and the only national charity dedicated to improving its diagnosis, prevention and treatment. Since 1986, the NOS has worked hard to raise public awareness and to offer support to people with osteoporosis, their families and carers through a range of information booklets, a national telephone helpline and a network of support groups.

The NOS raises awareness of bone health among people of all ages and fundraises for research into osteoporosis, to increase understanding of the disease and improve treatment options and patient care. Many people know what osteoporosis is, but few realise how serious it can be or that they are at personal risk.

For more information, visit www.nos.org.uk

## How to use this book

This book is made up of two parts. The first part concentrates on the importance of exercise for bone strength, and once you have read the introduction and realised the importance of exercise, turn to the section on Getting Started (page 20) and complete the questionnaires on pages 94–7, which will help you to select the exercises that are right for you.

Then, it's straight into the step-by-step programme of exercises to do at home. The last section 'Activities for Life' explores other types of exercises and activities that you can safely incorporate into your lifestyle to complement your strong bones workout.

The second part of the book focuses on a healthy diet for bone strength and offers over 120 delicious recipes for breakfasts, light snacks and soups, main meals and side dishes, puddings and cakes, all of which use bone-friendly ingredients.

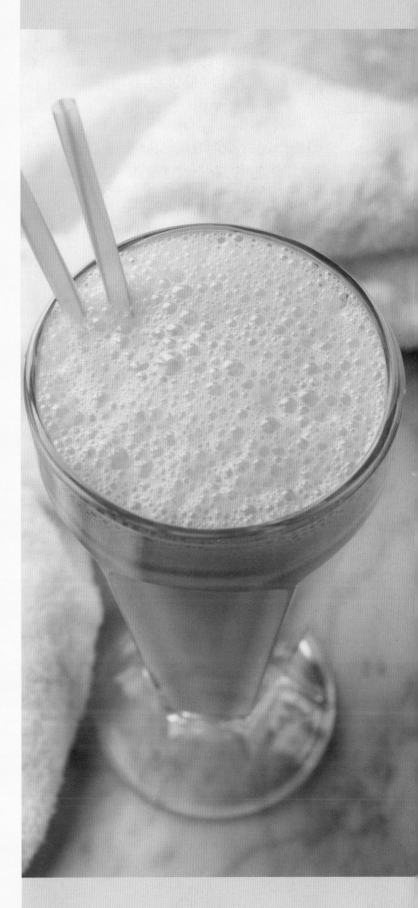

# WHAT IS OSTEOPOROSIS?

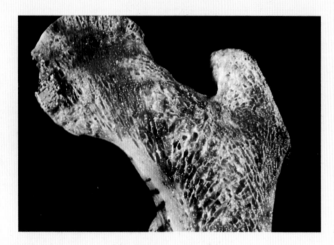

**Bone structure** *This is a cross-section of the top of a healthy femur showing solid outer bone and the honeycomb structure inside.*

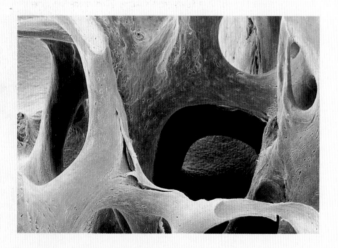

*This shows the honeycomb magnified. If a bone becomes osteoporotic, the walls of the honeycomb structure become thinner making the bone porous and fragile.*

Osteoporosis has been recognized as a problem, deserving of research attention and medical treatment, since about 1980. One in three women develop osteoporosis or 'brittle bone' disease. This means that bones break easily because the skeleton has become fragile.

Age-related osteoporosis is caused by gradual loss of bone mineral; this is a normal process, and is not a disease caused by infection. As bone mineral is lost, the bones do not shrink in size but become fragile and porous – the word 'osteoporosis' means porous bone.

From mid-life onward, the skeleton slowly loses bone mineral. If this bone loss is combined with less than average bone mineral density (BMD) before the menopause, then osteoporotic fractures become increasingly likely as the years go by. However, you can off-set this loss with exercise that stimulates increased bone formation, to improve your BMD. It is never too late to take steps to reduce your risk of fracture, by making sure your lifestyle includes small amounts of regular bone-friendly physical activity and a bone-friendly diet.

## The silent condition

Unfortunately, a fracture is often the first sign of osteoporosis. Osteoporotic fractures can occur very easily; changing a stiff gear in the car can be enough to break a brittle bone.

# UNDERSTANDING YOUR BONES

The bones that make up your skeleton are made from living tissue, which renews itself continuously throughout your life. If your skeleton is to do this effectively and remain strong, it needs regular stimulation from physical activities.

Bone is made of a calcium mineral, which gives bone its hardness and whiteness. This calcium mineral is embedded in a protein mesh of collagen, which is gristly and makes bone slightly bendy. Bone tissue is not completely solid, but has a honeycomb structure inside a thick solid outer layer. This efficient design maximises strength, without being too heavy.

The honeycomb structure of bone provides a huge surface area which is lined with bone cells. These cells continually renew the bone substance in a systematic cycle of breakdown and rebuilding, called bone turnover. This process ensures that minute fractures are repaired and the bone is kept strong. This remodelling allows bone to gain strength in response to increased load, or to lose it if loads become less.

## Key facts

★ Bones should be used regularly or they will deteriorate, like muscles do if they are not used.

★ The skeleton is a support structure that is alive and responds to challenging loads.

★ The normal 'loading' for the skeleton is the pull of working muscles on your bones and the force of gravity acting on your body weight. (Astronauts who live in a gravity-free environment lose bone density.)

★ Bones need a variety of brief, frequent loads every day to maintain their strength.

★ Bones need to be loaded a bit more than usual to improve their strength.

**Bone changes over time** *This graph shows how bone mineral density (BMD) falls with age. The middle line shows the BMD of an average woman over time, and the two outer lines show the BMD of an active and sedentary woman respectively. When BMD falls below the fracture threshold (when fracture becomes likely) a diagnosis of osteoporosis is made. The graph shows that this tends to happen at a much earlier age in sedentary women than in active women.*

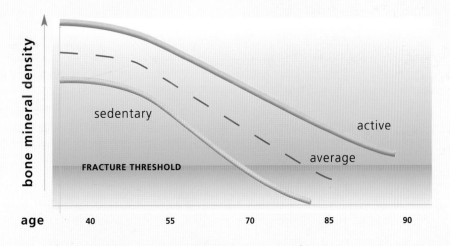

# HOW BONE CHANGES WITH AGE

During your early years, your body accumulates bone. Up to and during adolescence, bones grow rapidly. Most of your skeleton is in place by the end of your teenage years and the consolidation of the skeleton is complete by the time you are 30 years old. It is still possible, however, to achieve improvements in BMD after this age if you change from a sedentary lifestyle to a more active one.

Some women lose very little bone as they grow older but others can lose a lot, particularly in the first few years after the menopause because of the fall in oestrogen levels that occurs when menstruation ceases. The result is a loss of bone mineral over the next few years of up to five per cent each year.

Fortunately, this loss later slows down to a rate of about one per cent a year. Even so, the bone can eventually become so porous that fractures happen very easily. During the postmenopausal years, oestrogen levels are low, and vary from one woman to another. This variation in oestrogen levels may go some way toward explaining why some women are more vulnerable to osteoporosis than others.

**Exercise for everyone** *It is never too late or too early to take care of your bones; from the age of six to sixty, physical activity will benefit your skeleton.*

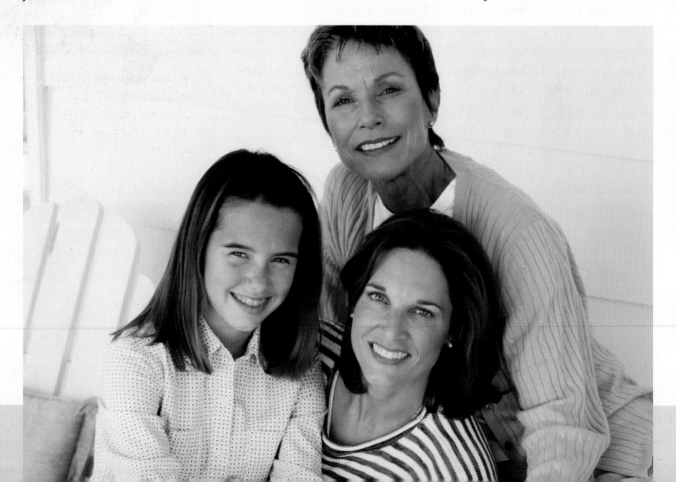

# ARE YOU AT RISK?

There are a number of factors that increase your risk of developing osteoporosis. Many of them are genetically programmed so you cannot do anything about them, but it does help to be forewarned. There are other factors you can do something about (see page 15). Your lifestyle is very important and you may need to change only a few aspects of your life to reduce your chances of developing osteoporosis. If you think you might be at risk, see your doctor to arrange a DXA bone scan and, if necessary, seek treatment to prevent fractures occurring later. The main risk factors which you cannot change are:

### GENDER
Women are at greater risk than men because they have smaller bones which contain less mineral. Oestrogen is important for bone health in women, and oestrogen levels fall at the menopause.

### FAMILY HISTORY
If you have relatives, particularly your mother or a grandmother, who have suffered from osteoporosis you are more likely to do so.

### BUILD
Small, slight women are at greater risk than large women, because they have smaller bones and lower BMD. Women of tall, thin build are also more vulnerable because of the long thin shape of the end of their hip bone. This is where almost half of all hip fractures occur.

### EARLY MENOPAUSE OR HYSTERECTOMY
Women who have stopped menstruating before 45 years of age or have had a hysterectomy (removal of the womb) before this age are at greater than average risk of developing osteoporosis. This is the case even if the ovaries were not removed. If you take hormone replacement therapy (HRT) from the time of the surgery, your risk of osteoporosis is reduced because the oestrogen is replaced but you are protected only for as long as you take HRT.

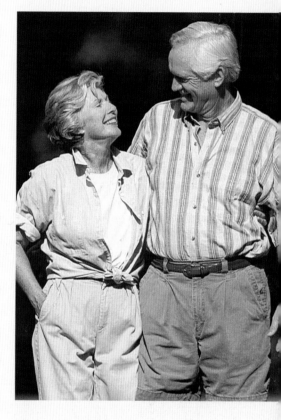

**The gender divide** *Women are more vulnerable to osteoporosis than men because their bones are smaller and the skeleton is not protected by testosterone.*

## ETHNIC GROUP

For genetic reasons, black women of African descent have a ten per cent lower risk of osteoporotic fracture than white women of Caucasian descent. Asian women are somewhere in between.

## THYROID PROBLEMS

Occasionally the thyroid gland becomes overactive, causing hyperactivity, or underactive, causing lethargy. It is difficult to adjust treatment to get the hormone levels exactly right. Too much thyroid hormone leads to some loss of bone density.

## STEROID TREATMENT

A number of diseases are treated or managed with cortico-steroids, including rheumatoid arthritis, Crohn's disease and severe asthma. Unfortunately, a common side effect is a weakening of the skeleton.

## GUT OR KIDNEY CONDITIONS

Diseases in which absorption of calcium is difficult or too much calcium is lost in the urine threaten calcium stores and lead to loss of bone.

## A HISTORY OF EATING DISORDERS

Failure to eat a normal, balanced diet by young women leads to bone loss which is associated with hormonal disturbances, loss of menstrual periods and extreme thinness. Diagnoses of osteoporosis can occur, therefore, in young women. Even after periods have resumed and body weight is back to normal, BMD may not return to previous levels. This loss of bone is likely to persist into middle age, leading to increased risk of fracture.

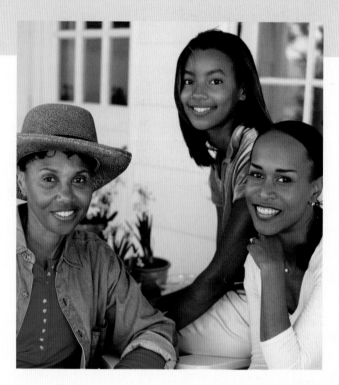

**Family matters** *You could be at a greater than average risk from osteoporosis if any other member of your family has a history of the condition.*

## Taking the pill

Whether oral contraceptives have any effect on bones is a common concern. Contraceptive pills are a form of HRT taken to override the natural pattern of hormonal release that leads to ovulation and potential pregnancy. They contain oestrogen and inhibit a woman's own oestrogen production. There is currently no evidence to show that taking oral contraception has long-term implications for the skeleton.

# THE WEAK SPOTS

The bones that are most likely to fracture due to osteoporosis are the wrist, spine and hip. Many of these fractures follow a fall, so maintaining good control of balance is important. You can live with fragile bones if you manage to avoid subjecting them to high impact.

### HIP

Fracture of the hip is a risk for women late in life which can cause a great deal of misery. Admission to hospital and major surgery to pin the broken ends of the bone together is often needed, and although this is usually a successful operation, many older victims never fully recover their mobility and independence.

### SPINE

Trying to force a stiff window or key can be enough to cause a fracture if your spine is osteoporotic. Signs that you might already have spinal osteoporosis are height loss and curvature of the spine (or 'Dowager's hump'). Once a vertebra has collapsed,

there is, at present, no way of rebuilding it. If several vertebrae collapse, the curvature of the spine can lead to health problems. For example, respiratory diseases can develop because there is not enough room in the chest.

### WRIST

The most common cause of a fractured wrist is when you reach out and use your hand to take the impact of a fall. A broken wrist is not a disaster but it can be very painful; it may not heal in exactly the right position and can cause long-term discomfort. A wrist fracture is a warning that you might have osteoporosis and that it is time to take action to prevent any more fractures occuring.

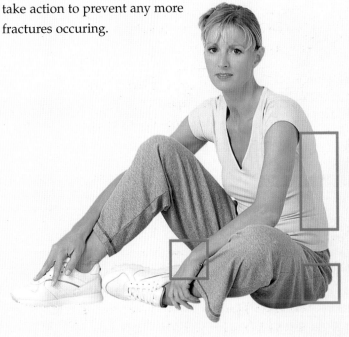

***Understanding your skeleton*** *Certain areas of the skeleton are more at risk from fracture due to osteoporosis, namely, the hip, spine and wrist.*

---

### Don't smoke

Smoking has been shown to increase the risk of fracture and the more cigarettes smoked each day, the greater the risk. If you smoke, then the best thing you can do for your bones is to give it up. Your skeleton will recover to some extent and your health will benefit in many ways. Try also to avoid passive smoking.

# PREVENTION & TREATMENT

If you think you may be at high risk of osteoporosis your doctor will probably send you for a scan. If you have been diagnosed with osteoporosis then there are a number of drugs that your doctor can prescribe. You will need to discuss the options with your doctor to determine which is right for you. These drugs work to reduce your risk of breaking a bone.

## THE IMPORTANCE OF EXERCISE
Whether you choose to take a drug treatment or not, you can further improve your BMD and reduce your fracture risk by making adjustments to your lifestyle. Research has shown that women who took part in regular exercise as well as starting HRT improved their BMD more than women who either exercised only or took HRT only.

*Improving bone strength* The exercises contained in this book have been shown to improve BMD if practised regularly. This exercise targets the hip (see page 52).

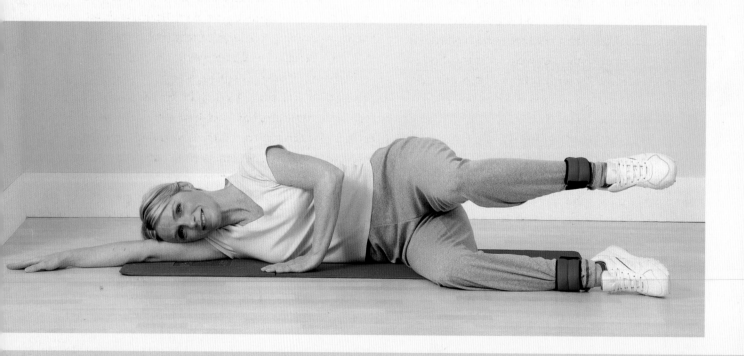

# REDUCING YOUR RISK

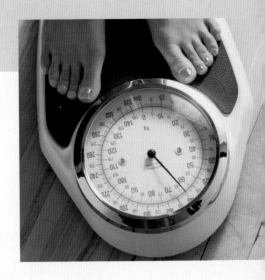

**Keep an eye on the scales** *The weight you carry is good for loading your bones, and any extra natural padding protects your bones from fracture if a fall occurs.*

There are several steps you can take to look after your bones and to ensure that you go into the menopause in the best possible health, steps that will also help maintain your BMD after the menopause.

## FEED YOUR BONES

A healthy diet, rich in calcium, vitamin D, and other vitamins and minerals is key to optimum bone health. The second part of this book outlines the nutritional steps you need to take and offers a wide selection of recipes that will help you achieve this.

## MAINTAIN A HEALTHY BODY WEIGHT

The bigger your bones are, the stronger they are, and the heavier you are, the denser your bones are, but this is not an excuse to eat too much! It is, however, very important to realise that dieting to lose weight is not good for your bones.

Weight loss has been associated with bone loss at all ages in adult life. Women who weigh more than 70 kg (11 stone) are unlikely to have an osteoporotic fracture, but if you are not tall there are health reasons why you should not weigh this much. If you are within the healthy weight limits for your height, you shouldn't go on a weight-loss diet unless your doctor recommends it.

## TAKE SOME EXERCISE

Active women have half the risk of fracture compared to those who do not take any exercise. Physical activity reduces the risk by improving both BMD and balance so that falls and fractures are less likely. Not all exercise is beneficial for your bones, however. Research has shown that the best exercise for your bones is brief bouts of activity that 'load' the skeleton.

## CHOOSING THE RIGHT EXERCISE

Endurance activities such as swimming or cycling are excellent forms of exercise for many reasons, but unfortunately they do not improve your bone health. Activities that provide a short sharp increase in skeletal loading are highly effective for your bones, provided they are more challenging than your normal activities (see page 96). The good news is that only a few loadings are needed to have an effect; about 50 per day. More than that does not achieve further improvement. This means that you can find time to improve your bone health without having to embark on a lengthy regimen. Regularly taking the stairs instead of the elevator might do it.

Just one minute of jumping or skipping (see pages 90–91) is useful, if it is right for you. It is important to realise, however, that these activities can prove dangerous for women with undiagnosed osteoporosis. They are therefore safe only for healthy premenopausal women.

Effective bone-loading depends on the force of gravity acting on your body and on any weight you lift, as well as the pull of muscles on your bones as you exercise. This can be achieved in many ways and the dynamic resistance exercises in the main section of this book are safe for everyone, including older women.

# GOOD PRACTICE

The next four pages contain advice that will help protect your spine and allow you to follow the exercises freely and safely.

## The importance of posture

Everyday activities at work or at home often lead us to spend far too much time hunched over. The result is poor posture, which increases tiredness and can place a strain on the spine. Good posture is essential for the health of the skeleton and for safe and effective movement in everyday life.

## Check your posture

Stand in front of a long mirror and compare yourself to the photographs below). Ask a friend to help with this. Check often when standing or sitting, to ensure that you have not slumped down.

## Improve your posture

* Lengthen your neck upward
* Ease your shoulders down
* Adjust your pelvic tilt
* Notice you have grown taller and slimmer

**Bad posture**

**Good posture**

*Bad and good posture* *When you adjust your posture so that your vertebrae sit properly, you feel and look taller and slimmer. The dotted line shows how much height you gain by correcting your posture.*

*Back of the neck long*

*Correct pelvic tilt*

*Chin parallel to the floor*

*Ribs lifted up from the hips*

*Abdominals tight*

*Knees soft*

*Weight distributed evenly*

## The importance of pelvic tilt

A correct pelvic tilt is an essential part of good posture. The difference between the correct and incorrect position of your pelvis is a subtle one, needing only a slight tightening of some muscles such as the abdominals, and a loosening of others in your lower back. The photographs (below) show you how to achieve it.

The effect of this slight but vital adjustment is to bring your spine into alignment. Your back will still have natural curves. It should feel good but it will need practice until it becomes an automatic part of

you. Do not let your abdominals tighten up so much that you cannot breathe properly.

All the exercises in the programme need to be performed with a correct pelvic tilt to ensure they are done safely, accurately and effectively.

### Tip

★ If you have stiff shoulders, start by shrugging your shoulders up to your ears before easing them down.

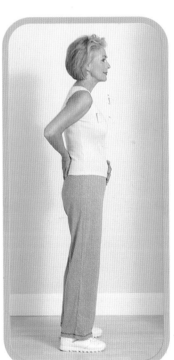

*1* Stand with your feet hip-width apart and your weight distributed evenly between both feet. Relax your shoulders and place your hands as shown.

*2* Stretch your spine upward as if someone is pulling the crown of your head upward. Tilt your pelvis so that your hips move up toward your face and your tail-bone moves down. Tighten your abdominal muscles to hold the tilt in place. Lift your chest and lengthen the back of your neck to further straighten the spine.

# LOOK AFTER YOUR BACK

Almost everyone gets back pain at some time in their lives and it can prevent them leading an active life. One of the most common causes of back pain is damage to the discs between the vertebrae, or a sprain of the back muscles or ligaments due to lifting something too heavy or lifting something in an awkward manner.

Lifting from the floor with your arms extended and your back bent is a recipe for disaster as the leverage is poor, so the weight borne by your back is perhaps ten times the weight you are trying to lift. If the muscles are not strong enough, the ligaments take too much strain and may tear. Using the lifting technique shown below will help you to protect your back; remember to use this technique for all lifting tasks.

Maintaining good posture throughout the day and using a chair that supports your lower back helps to prevent back pain. If you have a back problem or have had a hip fracture, you should avoid lifting heavy objects.

*1* Stand with your feet and legs hip-width apart, with one leg slightly forward. Bend your knees and keep your back straight.

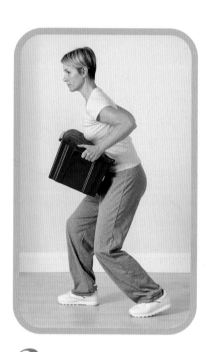

*Keep the object as close to your body as possible*

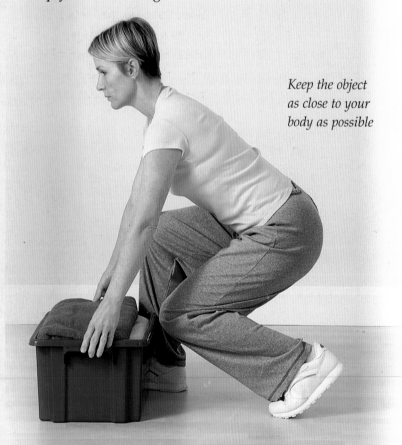

*2* Before lifting, check your pelvic tilt and tighten your abdominals. Bring the weight in toward your body. Stand up slowly, keep your back upright and make your legs do the work.

# STRENGTHEN YOUR PELVIC FLOOR MUSCLES

Many women become less active than they would like to be because they suffer from weak pelvic floor muscles. These muscles help control the bladder outlet and they are often weakened or damaged during childbirth. The embarrassing result of this is that urine leaks out easily. Like any muscles, pelvic floor muscles grow weaker with age but they will improve in strength if exercised regularly.

## Pelvic floor exercises

If you are out of practice with your pelvic floor muscles, you will need to rediscover them. Try the exercises seated to begin with. You will find the muscles easier to locate in this position and if the rest of your body is relaxed. When you have mastered the exercises you can do them any time, anywhere, as nobody but you will know what you are doing. If you have weak pelvic floor muscles, do both exercises four times a day until there is an improvement, then a minumum of once a day for maintenance.

*1* **Slow** Close, and draw up the back, then the front passages in your pelvic floor area as slowly and as strongly as you can, as if you were trying to prevent passing wind and urine. The feeling is one of 'squeeze in and lift up'. Hold for a count of 6, then release slowly, and with control. Repeat 4 times.

*2* **Fast** In one swift movement, tighten and lift both the back and front passages in the pelvic floor area. Hold for a count of one, then release slowly and with control. Repeat 6 times.

## Caution

★ Avoid tightening your abdominals or buttocks, squeezing your legs together or holding your breath.

★ Do not practise these exercises while urinating as this may cause infection.

# GETTING STARTED

This section sets out guidelines to ensure you get maximum benefit from the Home Exercises (see page 38) and the recommended Activities for Life (see page 82). The guidelines are linked to two questionnaires (see pages 94–7) which you must complete. These assess your current health and level of physical activity and will enable you to tailor your own exercise prescription. Everyone is different so it is important to choose the exercises that are right for you.

## Starting points

Everyone has different amounts of activity in their lives already. If you are regularly active you may need to add only one or two bone-specific exercises to your routine depending on what kind of exercise you are already doing. To get this right, find out where you are starting from with the physical activity questionnaire on page 96. If you are totally sedentary and unused to exercise, this book is for you too. The good practice section and these guidelines will enable you to tackle the Home Exercises one by one, sensibly and safely.

## Health issues

Some of the exercises will be more suitable for you than others, so before you start the programme, complete the health questionnaire on page 94. This will help you to select the most beneficial combination of exercises and makes it clear whether or not you should check with your doctor before getting started. This book has been written with healthy adult women aged up to 70 years in mind.

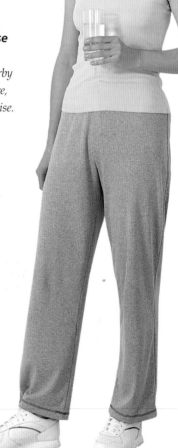

***Prepare for exercise***
*Have a glass of water (not coffee or tea) nearby so you can drink before, during and after exercise.*

## *Before you start*

★ Do not exercise on a day that you feel unwell or very tired.

★ Wear appropriate footwear and comfortable clothing, ideally cotton.

★ Ensure the room is clear of obstructions, not too hot or cold and well ventilated.

★ Make sure you will not be interrupted.

## Setting goals

We all need goals to keep us going. Think about what you want to achieve, plan your programme and chart your progress using the questionnaire on page 96. Your own motivation is essential. Your bones need regular exercise for the rest of your life, not over enthusiastic bursts of physical activity at sporadic intervals.

★ Set aside a specific time to exercise, depending on whether you are a morning or evening person, e.g. at 1.00 pm on Mondays, Wednesdays and Saturdays.

★ Make sure your programme will fit in with your daily life.

★ If you have not exercised for a long time, set yourself realistic goals and start at a leisurely pace.

★ Build up your programme over time, perhaps adding a new exercise once a month.

★ If you are very short of time, do some of the exercises once a week for maintenance; this is better than doing none at all.

## Listen to your body

It is important to appreciate the difference between working hard and overworking. If you are working effectively, you should be breathing a little more heavily than usual, feeling warm, perhaps sweating lightly and you should have a sensation of effort in your muscles.

Pain of any kind is a warning sign so never ignore or work through it. If any pain persists when you stop exercising, seek medical advice.

## Getting the most from exercise

★ Always warm up and cool down.

★ Take pride in using the correct technique.

★ Move with control and good posture.

★ Always work at your own level and progress cautiously.

★ Never exercise to the point of exhaustion.

★ Progress each exercise week by week to maintain the load on the skeleton and ensure you get an improvement.

★ Work through all the recommended stages of progression.

★ Avoid trying to beat the clock or another person. This programme is not about winning, it is about long-term benefit.

## Warning signs

★ Stop exercising and seek medical advice if you experience:
  Pain or discomfort
  Dizziness, faintness or nausea
  Shortness of breath
  Rapid heart rate
  Excessive sweating
  Sudden feeling of exhaustion
    or weakness

★ Slow down if you are:
  Feeling heavy limbed or shaky
  Breathing heavily
  Feeling overheated
  Losing concentration

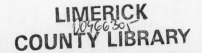

## Getting the load up

Most of the exercises depend on the resistance caused by the pull of gravity on your body mass. Some need the addition of weights or other simple equipment to increase the resistance. This is why we refer to 'weight-training'. Weights have advantages for bone-loading because of the stabilising muscle activity needed around the spine and hip and the variety of loading. However, they are potentially dangerous if dropped or if your lift gets out of control, so set an upper limit of 7 kg (15 lbs) for arm lifts and 11 kg (25 lbs) for leg lifts. Some exercises carry lower limits for safety; look for them under 'progression'. Take care when moving weights around. A few exercises require a partner; arranging to do them with a friend will help you to stick to your routine.

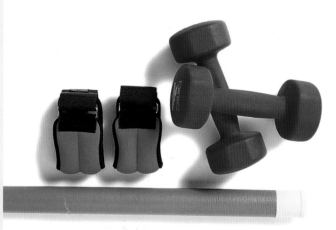

***Equipment to increase the resistance***
*Strap-on weights, dumb-bells, and body bars are available from all leading suppliers of exercise equipment. They come in graded sets from 500 g (1 lb) upwards.*

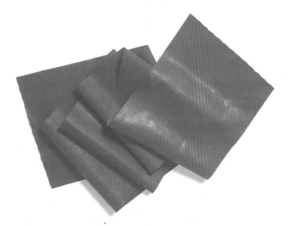

*Wide strips of strong rubber material, known as resistance bands, are also available in various colour-coded thicknesses. They give you a graded resistance to work against as you try to stretch them out.*

### Daily programme

★ Practise good posture and pelvic tilt throughout the day (see pages 16–17).

★ Do lots of pelvic floor exercises (see page 19).

★ Do one balance exercise. Vary them from day to day (see pages 40–45).

★ Go for a brisk five minute walk.

★ Climb a few flights of stairs.

★ Do some stretches (see pages 80–81).

### Weekly programme

★ Aim for three 40 minute sessions a week. Choose exercises that address your current needs from among the Home Exercises (see page 38) or the Activities for Life (see page 82). There are more suggestions on page 97.

★ You may wish to target your hip or wrist if you have below normal BMD at that site, so we have identified the specific benefits of each exercise in the Purpose boxes found on each page.

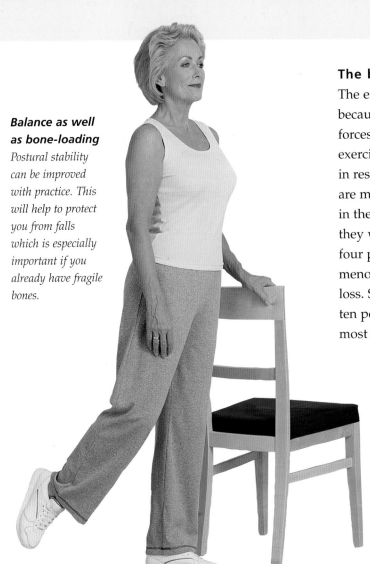

**Balance as well as bone-loading**
*Postural stability can be improved with practice. This will help to protect you from falls which is especially important if you already have fragile bones.*

## The benefits for bone

The exercises are effective for increasing BMD because they cause your muscles to generate large forces in the tendons which attach them to bone. The exercises have been chosen because they were found in research studies to benefit bone at the sites which are most liable to fracture. If you do these exercises in the way they are prescribed, three times a week, they will probably increase your BMD by three or four per cent over a year, and if you are post-menopausal, they will at least prevent further bone loss. Some women have shown increases of up to ten per cent and those with the lowest BMD are the most likely to benefit.

**Stretch and relaxation**
*Always rest in between bouts of exercise; there is no need to get out of breath or tired. Stretching after you have exercised is effective for keeping you supple.*

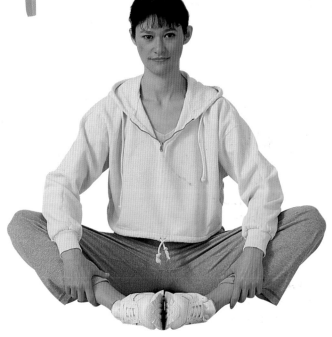

## Commitment

Bone changes slowly, so a long-term commitment is needed. Do a little exercise regularly and choose activities that you enjoy so that you will want to continue. Variety is good for your bones and helps to prevent boredom. Do not despair if the exercises take ages to do at first; you will get quicker with practice. Just like muscle, bone will deteriorate again if you stop exercising and your gains will slowly be lost.

# WARMING UP

The circulation, mobility and stretching exercises on the next few pages are essential preparation for the main programme. These gentle, rhythmic movements, mobilisers and held stretches get your muscles, joints and reflexes awake, loosened up, warm and ready for action. Stretching is especially important if you have been sitting for a while as your muscles may have become slightly stiff. Working through the warming up section will help to ensure that you do not injure yourself and you will find the main programme much more comfortable to perform.

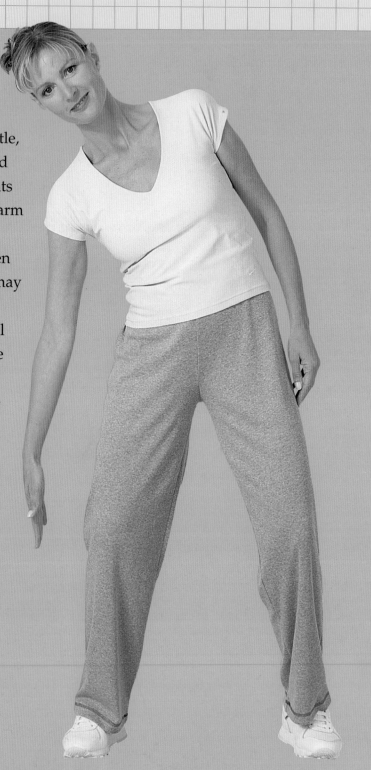

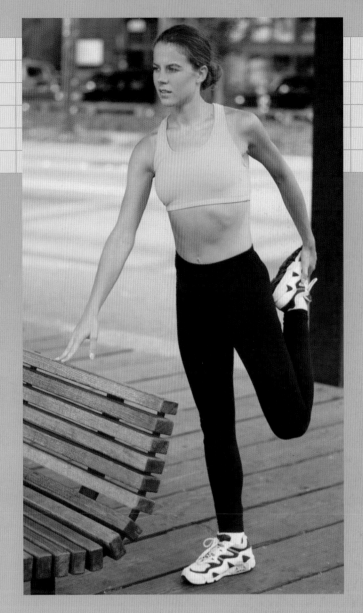

## THE BENEFITS OF WARMING UP

Muscles work most effectively when they are warm. They can generate more power and are stronger than when they are cold. Although you may not actually feel cold, your leg and arm muscles may be at a lower temperature than your trunk. For example, if you feel your calf muscle, you may find that the skin feels cooler than the skin on your neck. If you sit outdoors in cold weather, you may find that it is more difficult to walk when you stand up; this is because your leg muscles have been allowed to cool down in order to conserve heat for the rest of the body.

When you begin to exercise, it takes a few minutes before your blood flow increases and enough heat is generated to adjust your muscle temperature. You get hot when you exercise but only after you have been exercising for a while. The warming up exercises are designed to get your body ready before you start the main programme.

## *Safe exercise*

It is important that you complete all of the warming up exercises in the order given before moving on to the bone-loading exercises. It is also vital to cool down, especially after vigorous exercises such as running.

★ **Circulation** The first three exercises focus on the muscles, heart and circulatory system.

★ **Mobility** The next four exercises are designed to mobilise the joints.

★ **Stretching** The last six exercises stretch all the muscle groups that you will be using for the home exercises.

# WALK, SIDE-STEP & MARCH

This is the start of your programme so make it fun. Put on some lively music and enjoy the exercises. Starting your workout in this way can release tension, improve your focus and motivate you for the exercises to come.

Your movements should be gentle and your breathing should be steady. Build up the size and pace of your moves gradually; this allows the heart rate to increase steadily, making for safer and more effective exercise.

## *Purpose*

*Circulation exercises, sometimes referred to as pulse-raisers, are low-intensity, rhythmical activities that get the large muscle groups of your arms and legs moving to boost their supply of oxygen-rich blood and warm them up.*

### Adaptation
*To help you balance, you can perform the side-step exercise holding on to a chair.*

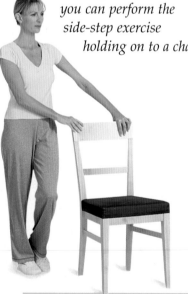

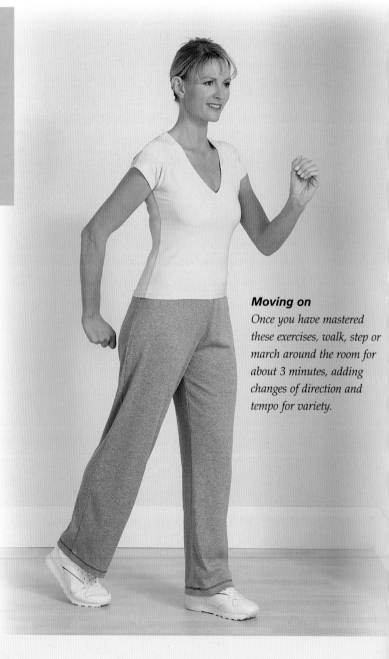

### Moving on
*Once you have mastered these exercises, walk, step or march around the room for about 3 minutes, adding changes of direction and tempo for variety.*

## *1* Walk

Check your pelvic tilt and tighten your abdominals. Walk on the spot, keeping your toes on the floor. Lift your arms with each step. Continue for 2 minutes.

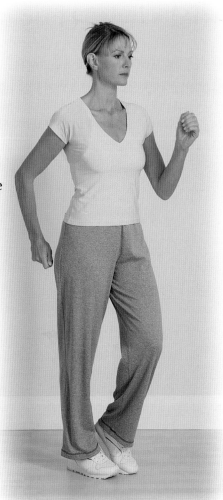

## *1* March

March gently on the spot, lifting the opposite arm to the lifted knee. Continue for 2 minutes.

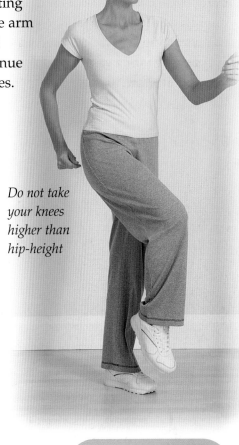

*Do not take your knees higher than hip-height*

## *1* Side-step

Step to the side, transferring your weight from the ball to the heel of your foot.

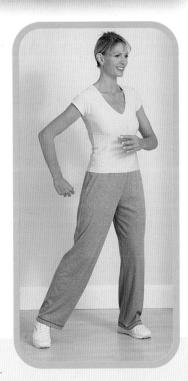

## *2* Bring your other foot in to touch the floor. Repeat to the other side. Swing your arms in the direction of the step. Continue for 2 minutes.

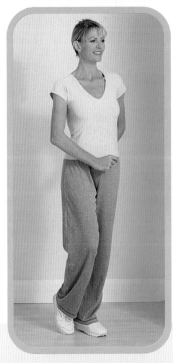

# SHOULDER & ANKLE MOBILISERS

To perform everyday actions with ease and comfort, freely moving shoulder joints are essential. Tasks such as reaching a high shelf or serving at tennis can be difficult if you have stiff shoulder joints.

Take time to explore your full range of movement in each direction. Move your shoulders forward, up, back and down. Stop if you feel any discomfort. Careful control and concentration on the quality of movement will improve your technique and increase your enjoyment and body-awareness.

When combined with good posture, this exercise can give your shoulder line and upper body a great shape. Slow shoulder circles are also a great way to release tension in the shoulder muscles.

Mobile, supple ankles ensure good balance, as the joints can respond better to uneven surfaces.

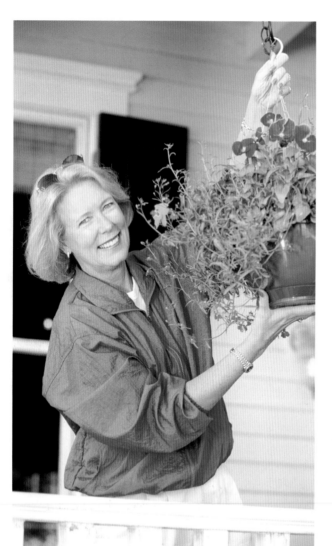

### Purpose

The shoulder exercise takes the shoulder joints slowly and smoothly through their full range of movement. This prepares them for the exercises to follow.

The ankle exercise helps to maintain the range of movement in the ankle joints and prepares them for the balance and resistance exercises.

**Stay strong and active**  *Supple shoulder joints and strong shoulder muscles are vital for maintaining your reach and allowing you to lift heavy items like this hanging basket from shoulder height.*

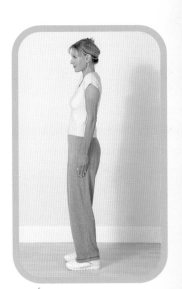

*Do not push out your chin*

*Avoid overarching your back*

*1* **Shoulder** Stand tall with your feet and legs a little wider than hip-width apart. Relax your shoulders and allow your arms to rest by your sides. Check your pelvic tilt and tighten your abdominals. Take both shoulders forward, then lift them up to your ears.

*2* Draw both shoulders backward in a large arc and ease them down and back away from your ears. Repeat up to 6 times.

## Common mistake

★ Avoid taking your feet too far apart as this reduces your range of movement in the ankle and puts unnecessary strain on the supporting leg.

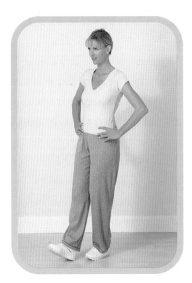

*1* **Ankle** Stand tall, check your pelvic tilt, and tighten your abdominals. Transfer your weight to one leg and place your other heel forward.

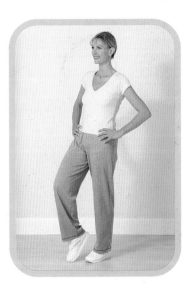

*2* Lift your front foot up by bending the knee and place your toes on the floor. Repeat this action 6 times. Repeat with the other foot.

# SIDE & TWIST: SPINE MOBILISERS

Mobility exercises stimulate the release of synovial fluid, the joints' natural 'oil'; this fluid nourishes, lubricates and protects your joint structures. These exercises also help to protect the vulnerable intervertebral discs.

A supple spine absorbs impact more efficiently than a stiff spine. Mobility exercises take the spinal joints through their full range of movement in two directions that are often neglected.

It is very important that you maintain a correct pelvic tilt for spinal exercises. Move slowly, fluently and with control. Extend the spine to its full natural range but never to the point of discomfort. Take a moment as you come back to centre each time to lengthen the spine and check your posture.

## *Purpose*

*These exercises help to mobilise the spine, maintain its range of movement and reduce the risk of back injury when you exercise.*

## Adaptation

*If you experience any pain in your lower back, or if you find it difficult to rotate without moving your hips, do the Twist exercise seated. Remember to do a pelvic tilt before you start.*

## *Caution*

★ Bear in mind that each individual's range of movement is different, so although you need to get your position as close to the pictures as possible, it is important that you find the movement comfortable.

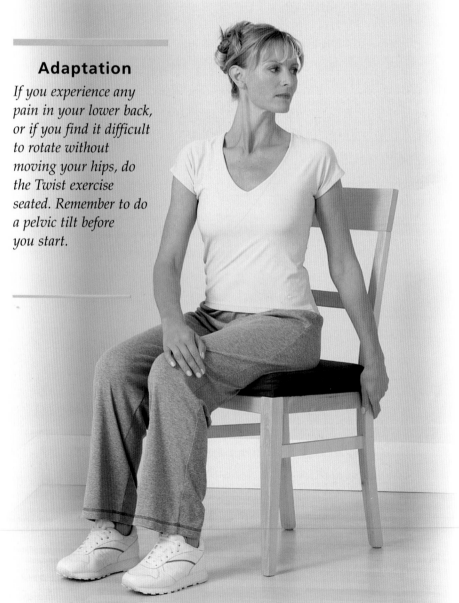

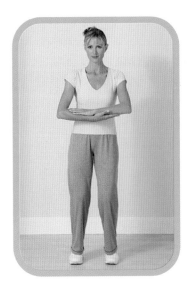

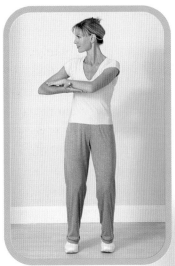

**2** Keeping your hips, knees and feet facing forward, lengthen your spine and slowly turn your upper body and head to one side, as far as you can. Return to centre, then repeat on the other side. Repeat up to 6 times.

**1 Twist** Stand tall with your feet and legs hip-width apart. Check your pelvic tilt, tighten your abdominals and bend both knees evenly. Hold your arms at chest height, resting one on top of the other.

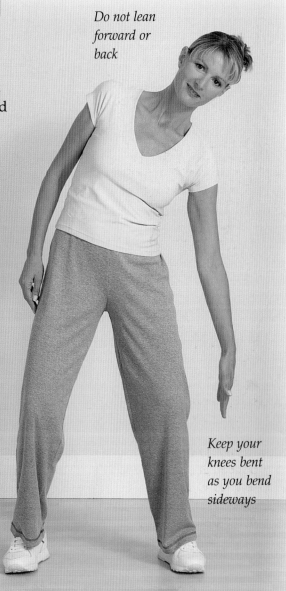

*Do not lean forward or back*

*Keep your knees bent as you bend sideways*

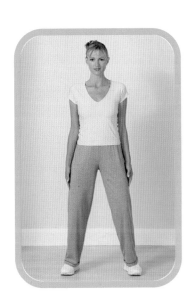

**1 Side** Stand tall with your feet and legs shoulder-width apart. Check your pelvic tilt, tighten your abdominals and bend both knees evenly.

**2** Lift up out of your hips, and bend slowly to one side, as far as your pelvic tilt will allow. Return to centre, then repeat on the other side. Repeat up to 6 times.

# CALF & THIGH STRETCHES

Muscles are adaptable and make themselves shorter over time if they are continually in a shortened position. This frequently happens to the calf muscle in women who do not wear flat shoes or walk barefoot. Such shortened calf muscles restrict ankle movements, but regular stretching reduces the stiffness and improves mobility.

Similarly, lengthening the quadriceps (the four muscles at the front of the thigh) through stretching improves the range of movement at the hip, transforms posture and so can help to prevent or alleviate back problems. Even if you have good posture, use a wall to support yourself, so you can focus fully on the quality of your stretch.

Stretching the quadriceps is one of the most important ways of counteracting the effects of prolonged sitting. Given today's sedentary lifestyles, both at work and home, this is a must for us all if we are to avoid becoming chair-shaped!

## Purpose

*These stretches prepare muscles for the exercises to follow and help to maintain the range of movement in the ankle and hip joints.*

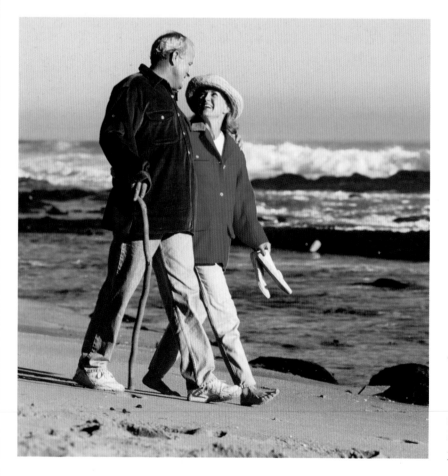

## Adaptation

*If you find balance difficult, use a chair to do the calf stretch. Keep your back straight, your chest lifted and pull your toe up toward your knee.*

**Walking barefoot**
*This is beneficial for the calf muscles and ankle mobility and helps to improve your balance, so take off your shoes whenever you can.*

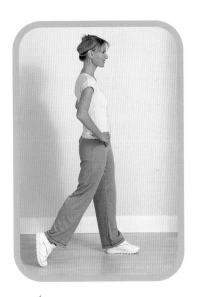

**2** Bend your front knee so that it is directly above your ankle. Press your back heel on to the floor and straighten this leg until you can feel a stretch in your calf. Hold for a count of 8. Repeat with the other leg.

*Lean slightly forward and upward to maintain a good body position*

**1** **Calf** Stand tall with your feet and legs hip-width apart and place your hands on your hips. Check your pelvic tilt and tighten your abdominals. Keeping your toes facing forward, take a stride backward with one foot and place it on the floor.

*Keep your back foot pointing forward*

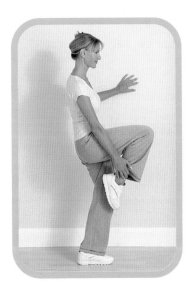

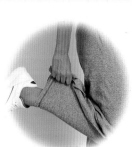

*If you have difficulty reaching your ankle, hold your sock or trouser leg*

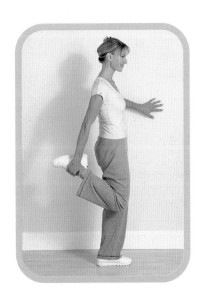

**1** **Thigh** Stand tall with a hand on a wall. Check your pelvic tilt, and lift your outer knee. Take hold of your ankle.

**2** Take your leg backward until your knee is just behind your hip. Straighten the supporting leg then increase your pelvic tilt and tighten your abdominals. Hold for a count of 8. Repeat with the other leg.

# SIDE & CHEST STRETCHES

*To stretch the muscles in the side of your torso and across the front of your chest. Both help to maintain good posture.*

Stretching the muscles at the side of your trunk helps to maintain spinal mobility and improve your posture. It is also good for releasing tension and this exercise will help maintain the range of movement in your shoulders. Always alternate sides when performing exercises that focus on the spine, as this gives a feeling of harmony and keeps the spine aligned and the body symmetrical.

Stretching the pectoral muscles across the front of the chest is an uplifting activity in every way. Most of us experience some rounding of the shoulders when sitting at a desk or because of poor posture and with this comes a sagging of the chest and restricted breathing. Pectoral stretches transform your posture as they lift the shoulders up and back and, in so doing, strengthen your upper back. This opens out your chest and allows for deeper breathing. The positioning of your arms needs particular care when doing the side stretch.

### Common mistake

★ Avoid reaching over too far without support; it can strain your spine.

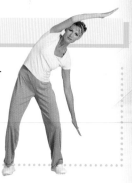

## Adaptation
*If balance is a problem, do the Side Stretch seated. Remember to check your pelvic tilt before you start.*

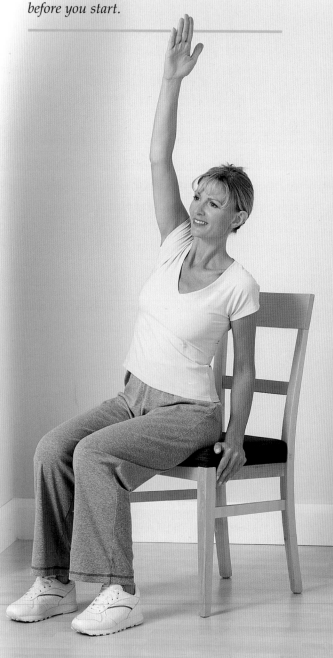

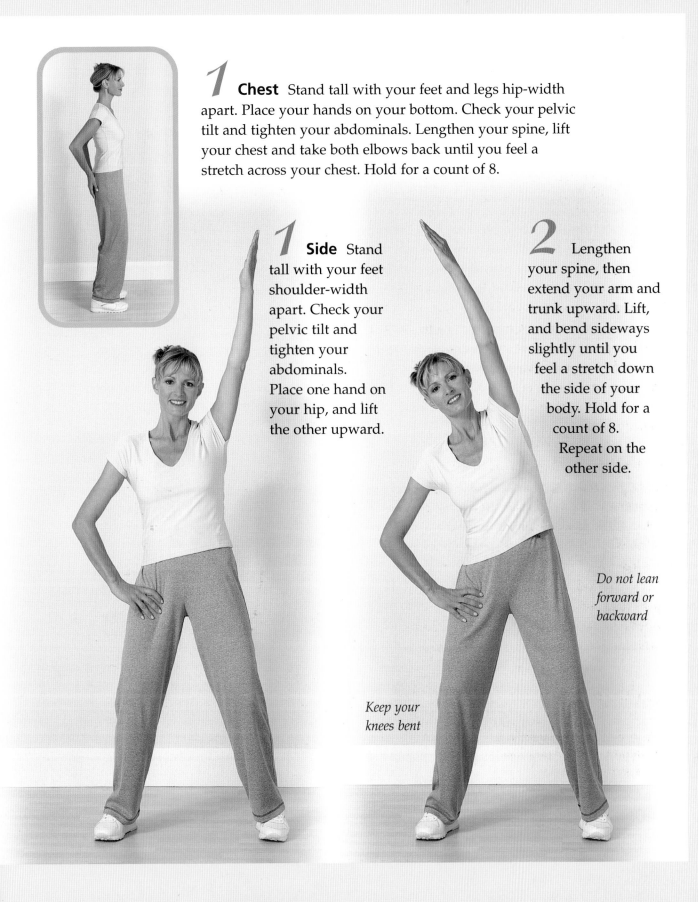

*1* **Chest** Stand tall with your feet and legs hip-width apart. Place your hands on your bottom. Check your pelvic tilt and tighten your abdominals. Lengthen your spine, lift your chest and take both elbows back until you feel a stretch across your chest. Hold for a count of 8.

*1* **Side** Stand tall with your feet shoulder-width apart. Check your pelvic tilt and tighten your abdominals. Place one hand on your hip, and lift the other upward.

*2* Lengthen your spine, then extend your arm and trunk upward. Lift, and bend sideways slightly until you feel a stretch down the side of your body. Hold for a count of 8. Repeat on the other side.

*Do not lean forward or backward*

*Keep your knees bent*

# HAMSTRING & TRICEP STRETCHES

The group of muscles located along the back of your thighs – the hamstrings – are among the most neglected muscles in the body, as well as those most compromised by an inactive lifestyle. Shortened, tight hamstrings can lead to restricted movement and back and hip problems, as well as an increased risk of injury.

The hamstrings may be notoriously tight muscles but they also respond well to attention and progress will be felt swiftly. Stretching these muscles can give you a new lease of life as many actions become that much easier.

The triceps muscles are located along the back of your arm. Stretching them will ensure suppleness in the shoulder joints so that upward reaching movements can be managed with ease.

## *Purpose*

*To stretch the muscles at the back of the thigh and to maintain range of movement in the hip and lower back.*

*To stretch the muscles at the back of the arm and to maintain range of movement in the shoulder joints.*

## *Caution*

★ If you have a history of falls or persistent balance problems, use a chair for support for these stretches.

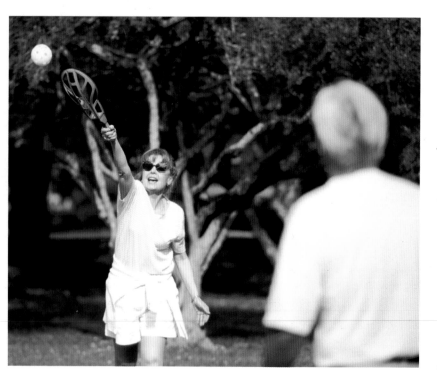

### Adaptation

*If you find the standing hamstring stretch uncomfortable, you can do this stretch seated. Keep your back straight and lean forward and upward to increase the stretch.*

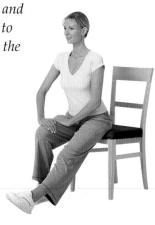

*Keep your chest lifted*

*Ensure your hips are level as you stretch*

## *1* Hamstring

Stand tall with your feet and legs hip-width apart. Check your pelvic tilt and tighten your abdominals. Lengthen your spine and transfer your weight to one leg. Slide your other foot forward, keeping your foot on the floor.

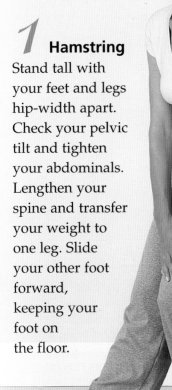

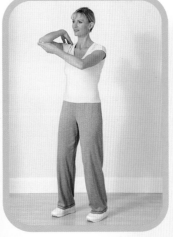

## *1* Tricep Stand

tall as before with your knees bent slightly. Place one hand on your shoulder and take the other arm across your chest. Check your pelvic tilt and tighten your abdominals.

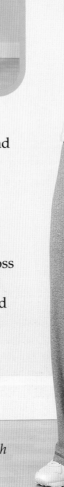

*Keep the spine and neck long*

*Do not overarch your back*

## *2*

Place both hands at the top of your weighted leg. Bend this knee as you bend forward from the hips until you feel a stretch in the back of your straight leg. Hold for a count of 8. Repeat with the other leg.

## *2*

Ease your raised arm up and back until you feel a stretch in your underarm. Aim to get the fingertips of your raised arm between your shoulder blades. Hold for a count of 8. Repeat with the other arm.

# HOME EXERCISES

This is a series of back, leg and arm exercises to load your skeleton in ways that should optimise your BMD. There are also balance exercises to help reduce your risk of falls. Between them these exercises will reduce your risk of fracture. The left-hand pages include cautions for your safety and advice about how to progress. The right-hand pages give detailed step-by-step instructions for each exercise. Invest time at the beginning paying careful attention to these instructions so that you master the correct technique and become competent quickly. With each new exercise, allow two sessions to learn the movement pattern, using the easiest alternative, before you begin to train in earnest.

Some of the bone loading exercises form complete packages, which have been evaluated as such in research trials; they may be effective only if practised together. One package is the first six leg exercises (pages 50–61) and the other package is the Arm Press (page 68), All-fours (page 74), and the Wrist Press, Twist & Pull (page 76).

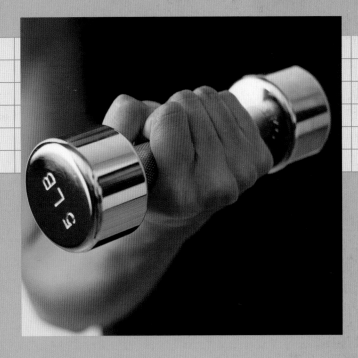

## A WORK-OUT FOR YOUR BONES

For improvement in BMD with weight-training, you need to lift at least 70 per cent of your maximum. This level is best tested in a gym (see page 89) but you can judge it at home from the effort you apply. If the eighth lift is easy you're below 70 per cent; if you can only just manage the last few lifts, you're above 80. You should train three times a week.

For maintenance of bone strength, continue to train once a week at the level you achieved. This should at least prevent further bone loss, which is a benefit if you are postmenopausal because these years are associated with progressive bone loss.

When you are ready to use weights:
★ Begin with 500 g (1 lb)
★ Progress in 500 g (1 lb) stages
★ Use no more than 7 kg (15 lbs) for arm lifts
★ Use no more than 11.5 kg (25 lbs) for leg lifts
Free weights are hard to control so the upper limits are set for safety not as a maximum for bone-loading. A larger woman will be able to lift more than a smaller one so we cannot prescribe a maximum. Few women will reach the safety limits, but if you do, then progress to a gymnasium and use the weight stacks, which allow you to use bigger weights with safety (see pages 88–9). Always move slowly, especially as you lower; you are more powerful when you move slowly and this will load the bones better.

Lift on the right and left sides in turn for the leg exercises (except the side leg lift and the leg press). If you are using weights, put one on each limb before you begin the exercise. Remember to follow the Essentials (*right*).

## Essentials

★ For each exercise aim to do 8 lifts, resting for a second between each lift.

★ Train up to 3 sets of 8 lifts (24 lifts in total), resting for a minute between each set.

★ Do not hold your breath; slowly count out loud to 3 as you lift (hold for a second) and count to 3 as you lower.

★ When the 8th lift is no longer a challenge, it is time to progress.

★ Aim to progress every 2 weeks.

★ If you have to stop due to illness, start again with less weight.

★ Stop if you feel any pain and reduce the weight.

★ Do not overtrain; up to an hour every other day is enough.

# FLAMINGO SWING

Good balance is important because if you lose your balance and fall, you might break any fragile bones. Taking steps to improve your balance is therefore a useful way of reducing the risk of osteoporotic fracture as you grow older.

We all have the potential to achieve excellent balance. Gymnasts, tightrope walkers and ice skaters are shining examples of what is possible with practice. You can train yourself to have better balance by practising Flamingo Swings. This balance exercise can enhance your control and flow of movement and sharpen the reflexes that help to prevent a trip from turning into a fall. Take the opportunity to practise them whenever possible, perhaps while you are waiting for the bus or talking on the telephone.

## Balance test

Keep a record of how long you can remain standing on one leg, even if it is only a second or two, and follow your improvement week-by-week until you can hold the position for 30 seconds.

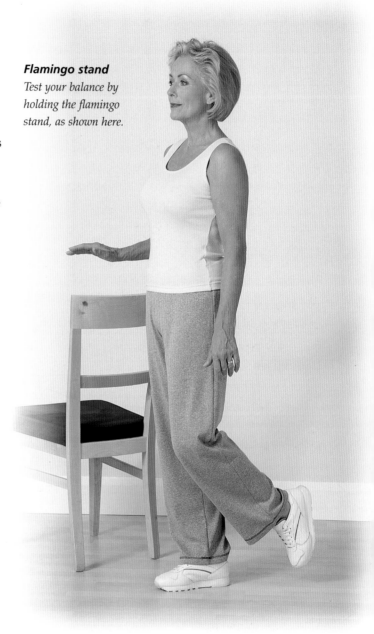

**Flamingo stand**
*Test your balance by holding the flamingo stand, as shown here.*

### Purpose

*This exercise improves balance and will reduce your risk of falls and fractures.*

### Caution

★  If you have a history of falls or persistent balance problems, use two chairs, one either side of you, for support.

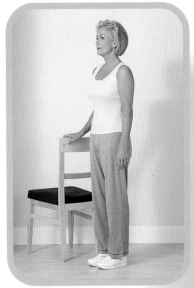

**3** Keeping both knees soft, swing the extended leg gently backward in a controlled sweeping motion, keeping it close to your body.

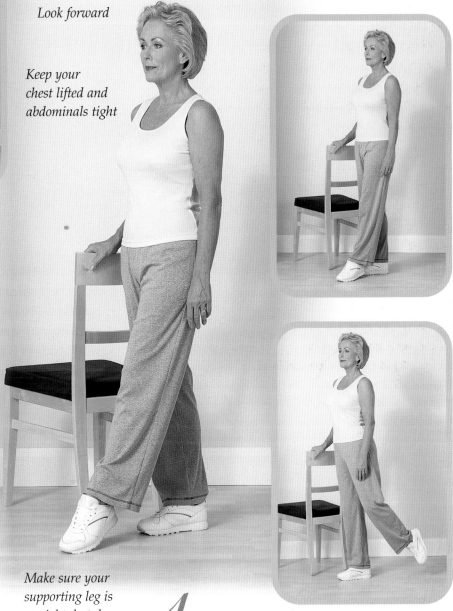

*Look forward*

*Keep your chest lifted and abdominals tight*

**1** Stand sideways to a chair, holding the chair-back for support. Stand tall, with your feet slightly apart and your weight distributed evenly between both feet. Relax your other arm by your side. Check your pelvic tilt and lift up out of your hips.

**2** Transfer your weight on to the leg nearest to the chair. Slide your other foot forward, keeping your toes in contact with the floor. Lift the extended leg about 5 cm off the floor.

*Make sure your supporting leg is straight, but do not 'lock' your knee*

**4** Keep both hips facing forward as you swing your leg forward. Do not allow your back to arch. Repeat 6 times. Turn and repeat on the other leg.

# TANDEM STAND & WALKS

Your feet form a very small base upon which to balance your body. Successful balance requires a continuous flow of signals through the nervous system from all over the body, from the soles of your feet, eyes, middle ear, muscles and joints.
In a Tandem Stand or Tandem Walk, the feet are placed in line, toe to heel, instead of side by side. Standing and walking on a narrower base than usual challenges the body to 'fine tune' its response system.

## Progression

Test your balance with a Tandem Stand. Once you can hold the position securely for ten seconds beside a wall, with both right or left leg forward in succession, progress to the Tandem Walk exercise to improve your balance.

**Advanced alternative**
*When you feel steady, perform the Tandem Walks without using the wall. Outstretch your arms to help you balance.*

### Purpose
*This exercise improves balance and stability and will reduce your risk of falls and fractures.*

### Caution

★ If you have a history of falls or persistent balance problems, use two chairs, one on either side, for support.

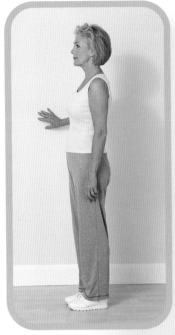

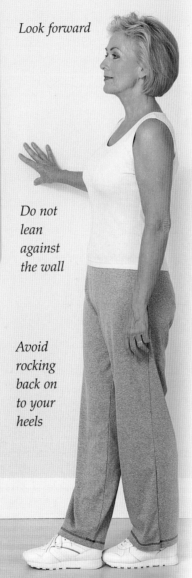

*Look forward*

*Do not lean against the wall*

*Avoid rocking back on to your heels*

## 1 Tandem stand

Stand sideways to a wall and place one hand on the wall for support. Relax your other arm by your side. Stand tall, check your pelvic tilt and tighten your abdominals.

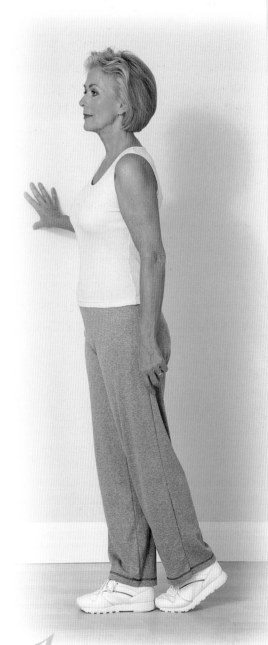

### Caution

★ Take care not to let your back toe catch on the heel in front. Avoid turning too quickly, and take small steps to turn around.

## 2
Place the foot nearest the wall directly in front of the other so your feet form a straight line. Hold for 10 seconds. Repeat with your other foot in front. Turn to face the other direction and repeat steps 1 and 2.

## 1 Tandem walk
Use a wall for support. Place one foot directly in front of the other so your feet form a straight line. Develop this movement into continuous walking. Take 10 steps, turn slowly and repeat in the other direction.

# TOE WALKS

### Purpose

This exercise improves your balance when moving. It is also good for improving calf strength and ankle flexibility.

These Toe Walks in combination with the Flamingo Swings and Tandem Walks provide comprehensive balance training and, if practised regularly, will reduce your risk of falls.

When you decide to get up and walk across the room, all the right messages go to all the right muscles in just the right order. As you grow older, however, small changes to the nervous system begin to make the challenge of maintaining effective postural control more difficult, eyesight becomes less sharp and coordination slows a little. It is, therefore, increasingly important that you practise good balance as you grow older.

**Progression**

When you feel secure enough, you can train your balance further by doing this exercise without using a wall for support. Put your hands on your hips to start with, then raise your hands above your head for a further challenge.

## Caution

★ If you feel unsteady, lower your heels to the floor. Rest, then begin again.

★ If you have bunions, or other foot problems that make this exercise difficult just practise Step 2, lifting your heels as much as you can. Use a chair in front for support.

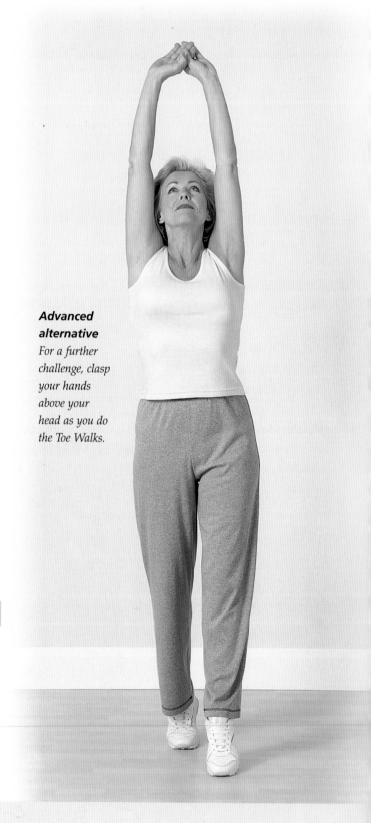

**Advanced alternative**
*For a further challenge, clasp your hands above your head as you do the Toe Walks.*

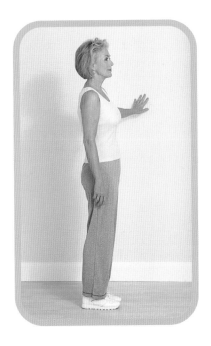

*1* Stand sideways to a wall, and place one hand on the wall for support. Relax your other arm by your side. Stand tall and check your pelvic tilt.

*Look forward*

*Keep your spine long, and your chest lifted throughout*

*3* Using the wall as support, walk 10 steps on your toes. Then bring both feet together by stepping in with your back foot. Lower your heels to the ground and turn around. Rise on to your toes and walk 10 steps in the other direction. Turn and repeat.

*Keep your abdominals tight and your weight distributed evenly over both feet*

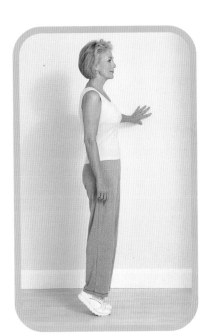

*2* Lift your heels and transfer your body weight on to the balls of your feet.

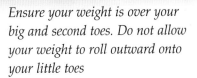

*Ensure your weight is over your big and second toes. Do not allow your weight to roll outward onto your little toes*

# BACK LIFT

This exercise targets the muscles running the length of the spine (erector spinae). As their name suggests, these muscles enable you to stand erect by supporting the length of the spine.

A sedentary lifestyle does not provide sufficient action for back muscles. They are rarely exerted strongly or often enough to maintain optimum strength, so unexpected demands can cause trouble. When inadequate strength meets too large a force, damage occurs to ligaments and tendons and the consequence is back pain. This is such a common problem that almost everyone has suffered from it at some time. Lifting a lively child or moving a heavy object can damage your back if it is not strong enough. If you have a history of back pain consult your doctor before starting and begin with the arm supported alternative shown in the adaptations.

**Progression**

Begin by lifting 5 cm (2 in), and progress to 10 cm (4 in). To go further, add a small flat weight across your shoulders. (The safety limit is 7 kg (15 lbs).)

### *Purpose*

To strengthen your back muscles, improve your spinal alignment and reduce the risk of vertebral fracture.

### *Caution*

★  If your lower back hurts during this exercise, place a folded towel under your hips. Do only two lifts and see how your back feels during and after the exercise. If there is any discomfort try the adaptations below until your strength improves. If pain persists, stop and consult your doctor.

★ If you are unable to get down to the floor safely, you can do this exercise in bed.

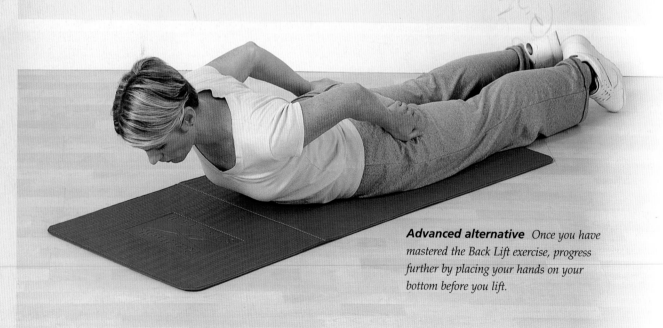

**Advanced alternative**  *Once you have mastered the Back Lift exercise, progress further by placing your hands on your bottom before you lift.*

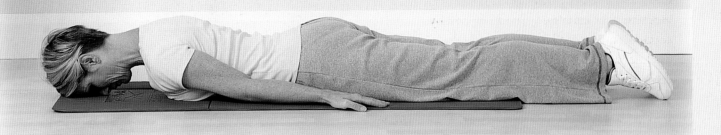

*1* Lie face-down on the floor, your legs together, your arms by your side and your palms on the floor. Check your pelvic tilt.

*Keep the back of your neck long and your eyes looking down*

*Make sure your feet stay on the floor*

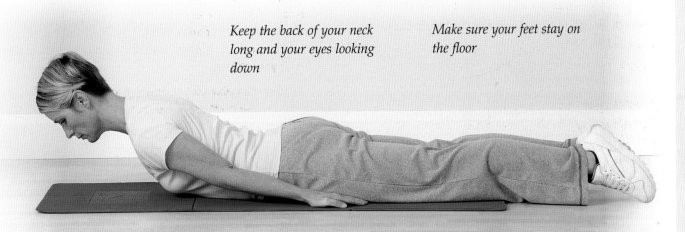

*2* Lengthen your spine and lift your shoulders, back and head off the floor. Moving slowly and with control, count to 5 to lift, hold, count to 5 to lower. Rest for 5 before repeating. Lift your palms just off the floor for an extra challenge.

## Adaptations

*Start by placing your hands, palms down, under your forehead, with your elbows bent comfortably to either side. Lift and lower as for the main exercise.*

*Progress by placing your hands, palms down, in front of you, with your elbows under your shoulders 'like a lion'. Lift and lower as before.*

# FLYING BACK LIFT

This exercise targets many muscles especially those running the length of the spine. It is a progression of the Back Lift (see page 46) and Leg Lift (see page 50) and you should do it only when you are comfortable with the Back Lift. It will improve your shoulder flexibility and strengthen the muscles that protect your shoulder joints. This helps to prevent 'frozen shoulder'; a painful condition that is common in older women. It also creates a satisfying sense of top-to-toe body line and improves body awareness and postural control.

**Progression**
When you have mastered the Flying Back Lift, progress by lifting your arm and leg higher, to a maximum of 10 cm (4 in).

## Purpose
To strengthen the muscles supporting the spine and the back of the hip, thigh, shoulder and arm, and reduce the risk of vertebral fracture.

**Advanced alternative** *Progress further by taking both your arms in a slow, controlled arc movement. As for the Back Lift, count to five while you complete the arc movement.*

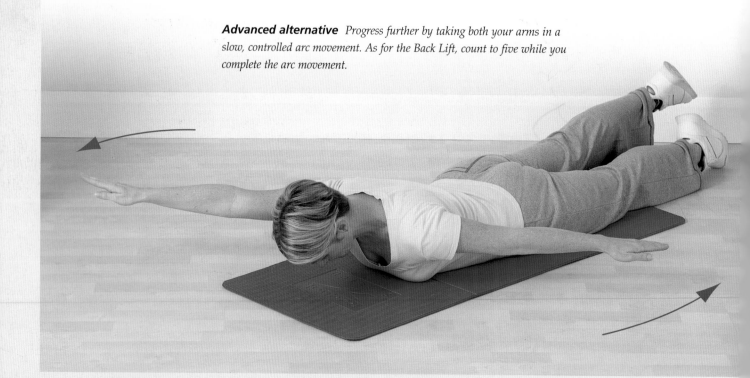

*Keep the back of your neck long, your chin in and your shoulders down throughout*

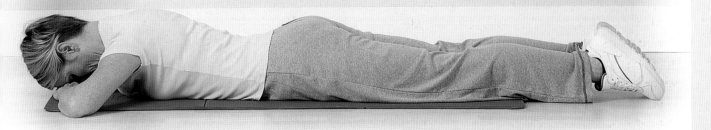

**1** Lie face-down with your forehead on your folded hands. Check your pelvic tilt and tighten your abdominals.

**2** Slide one palm forward along the ground. Lengthen your opposite leg along the floor away from your body.

*Avoid overarching your back; keep looking at the floor*

*Lengthen your leg as you lift*

*Keep your non-active foot in contact with the floor*

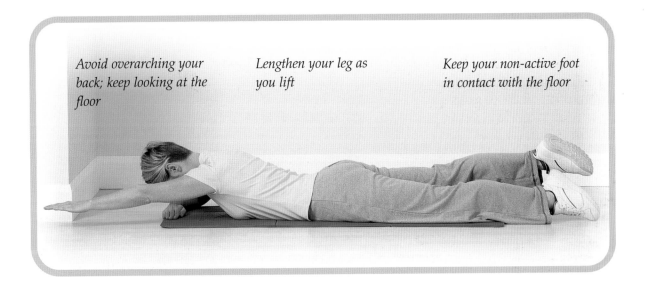

**3** Tighten your buttock muscles on this side, then lift your leg about 5 cm off the floor. Maintain this position as you lengthen and lift your outstretched arm about 3 cm. Count to 5 to lift, hold and count to 5 to lower. Rest, then repeat on the other side.

# LEG LIFT

## Purpose

To improve bone mineral density (BMD) and range of movement in the hip and spine. It also helps to strengthen the lower back, buttocks and the back of the thighs.

This exercise targets the lower back, buttocks and the back of the thighs (hamstrings). As you lift your leg, the muscles contract and pull on the bones of your spine and hip, which has a stimulating effect on BMD. It is also an excellent exercise for improving lower back strength, increasing the support for your lower spine and reducing the risk of lower back pain. It will also firm up the muscles of your bottom to give you a trimmer figure. These muscles are used in all weight-bearing activities but are only challenged to their full potential during vigorous activities such as uphill running or climbing up stairs quickly.

## Progression

When you have mastered the Leg Lift exercise, increase the challenge by using ankle weights.

## Caution

★ If you feel pain in your lower back during this exercise, place a folded towel under your hips to stabilise the pelvis and reduce the arch in your lower back. If the pain persists, omit this exercise and seek advice from your doctor.

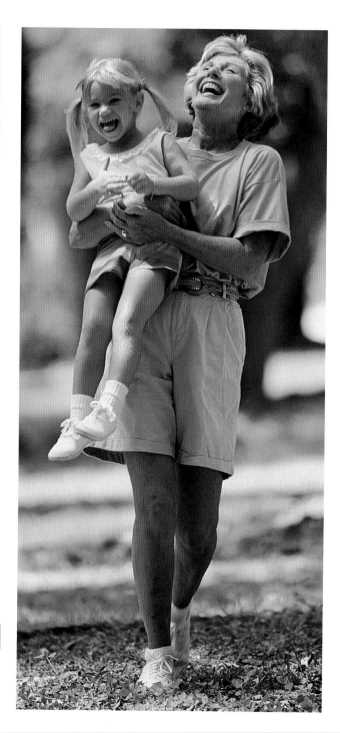

**An active life** *As you lift a child you use a wide range of muscles, including those in your lower back. Keeping strong will enable you to lead an active life, while minimising risk of injury.*

**1** Lie face-down with your legs together and your forehead on your folded hands. Check your pelvic tilt and tighten your abdominals.

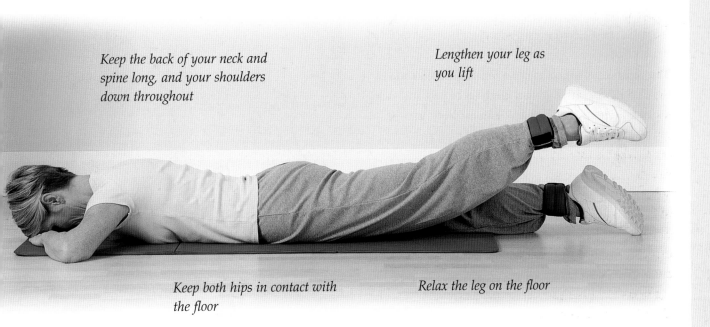

*Keep the back of your neck and spine long, and your shoulders down throughout*

*Lengthen your leg as you lift*

*Keep both hips in contact with the floor*

*Relax the leg on the floor*

**2** Lengthen one leg away from you along the floor, tighten your buttock muscles on this side and, keeping both hips pressed into the floor, lift your leg about 3 cm. Lengthen and lift another 3 cm upward, then lower. Count to 3 to lift, hold, count to 3 to lower. Rest, then repeat on the other side.

### Common mistake

★ Do not lift your leg so high that your hip lifts off the floor. This can place strain on your back.

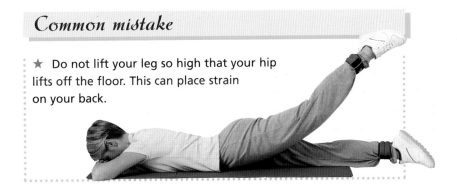

# Side Leg Lift

This exercise targets the large outer thigh muscles (the abductors), which are attached across the top of the femur to the outer edges of the pelvic girdle. These muscles are used when you step sideways but are rarely used to their full potential. If you make them work against some resistance, such as in this exercise, the underlying bone is stimulated.

### Progression

Start without weights and with bent knees. Add a light weight around your thigh to progress and then move the weight to your ankle to further increase the resistance.

### Purpose

To increase bone mineral density (BMD) in the hip. It also strengthens the muscles on the outside of the hip and thigh.

### Caution

★ If you have an artificial hip, start and finish with your knees bent and a cushion between your thighs.

**Advanced alternative** *Progress further by lifting with your top leg straight.*

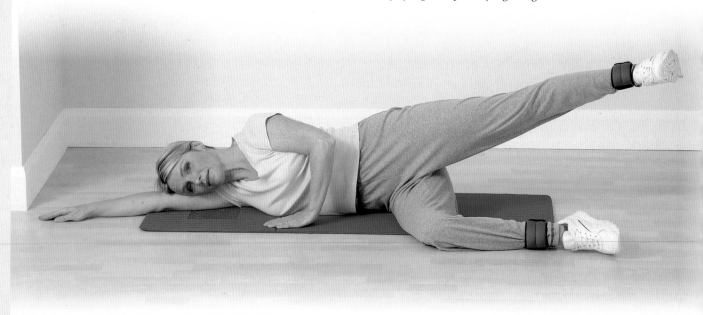

*Ensure your hips, trunk and shoulders are in a straight line*

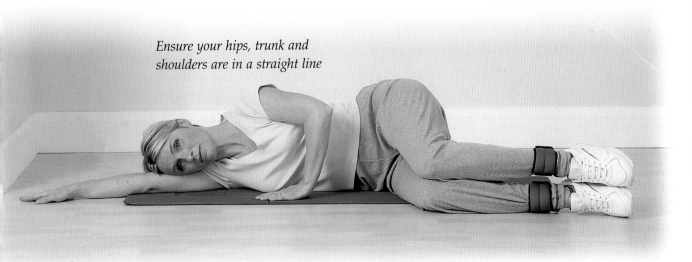

**1** Lie sideways with your knees and hips at right angles, with weights around your ankles. Rest your head on your lower arm or a cushion for comfort. Place your other hand on the mat, opposite your chest. Check your pelvic tilt and tighten your abdominals.

*Take care not to let your top hip and knee roll back*

*Keep your knee and ankle at the same height*

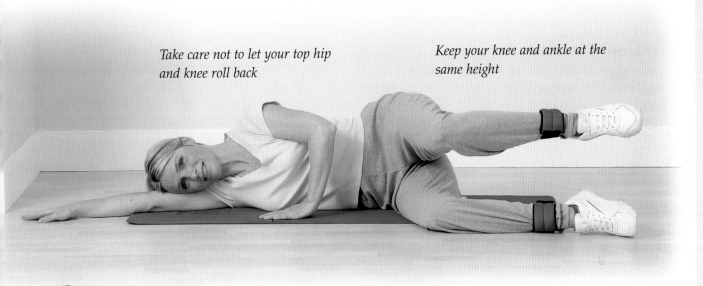

**2** Taking care to keep your knee and foot facing forward and slightly down, raise your top leg about 10 cm. Count to 3 to lift, hold, count to 3 to lower. Rest, then repeat. Roll over on to your other side and repeat with your other leg.

# THIGH SQUEEZE

## *Purpose*

To increase bone mineral density (BMD) in the hip. It also strengthens the muscles on the inside of the thigh.

## *Caution*

★ If you experience any pain in your pubic area or lower back, check your pelvic tilt and move a little further away from your partner. If the pain persists, stop, and try doing the exercise on your own using a resistance ball.

This exercise targets the inner thigh muscles (adductors), which pull the legs together. You use these muscles when horse-riding or swimming breaststroke, but on the whole, hip adduction is an unusual activity in everyday life. Exercising these muscles provides unusual forces for the underlying skeleton to resist, which is why it helps to improve the density in the hip.

Although swimming is a healthy activity, the forces are not high enough to stimulate bone. This is because the water yields as you kick. To load your bones, you need to work against a bigger resistance. A resistance ball is ideal, but it is fun and effective if you can work with a partner. It is important to choose a partner of similar size and strength to yourself. The added advantage is that while you are exercising your adductors, your partner is exercising her abductors (the outer thigh muscles), and vice versa when you change over.

**Progression**

Just squeeze as hard as you can.

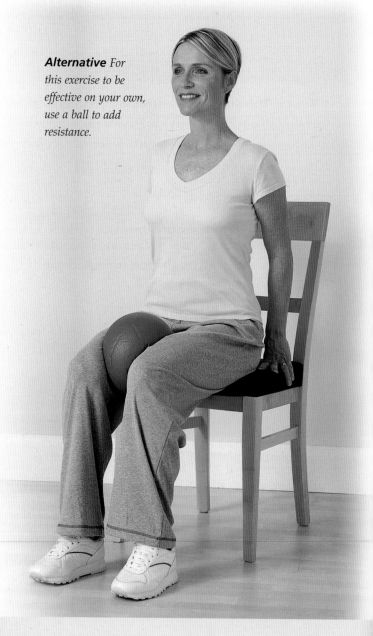

**Alternative** *For this exercise to be effective on your own, use a ball to add resistance.*

*1* Sit tall facing a partner, with your legs outside her legs. Both of you must position your knees directly over your toes, check your pelvic tilt and tighten your abdominals.

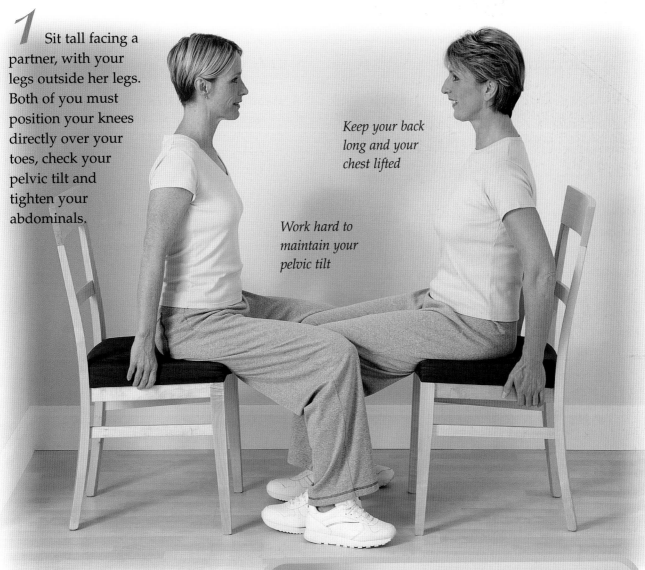

*Keep your back long and your chest lifted*

*Work hard to maintain your pelvic tilt*

*2* Slowly press your legs inwards, as your partner presses outwards. Count to 3 as you press, hold, count to 3 to release. Rest, then repeat.

*3* Rest, then change positions and repeat.

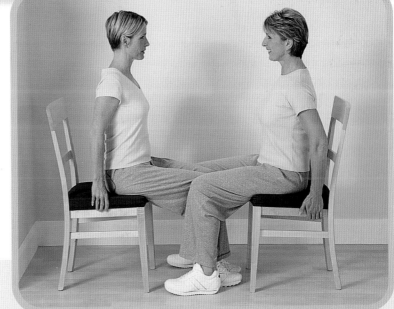

# LEG PRESS

### Purpose
To load the hip bone and strengthen the muscles at the front and back of the hips, thighs and knees.

### Caution

★ If you have knee problems take care not to lock your knees.

★ If you have an artificial hip do not lift the thigh into the chest; begin with the knee at hip height.

This exercise targets the muscles that straighten the hip, including the quadriceps, so it is good for increasing BMD in these areas. You use these muscles when you push off against the floor to rise from a chair or climb stairs. Activities like jogging and jumping also challenge these muscles and, in turn, promote BMD.

It is difficult to provide enough resistance in a home exercise for this group of muscles. You need to use both arms to provide resistance for one leg; if you still find it easy to stretch out the strongest band, use a weight-training machine in a gym to provide sufficient resistance. You will be surprised at how much you can push with your legs; these muscles can resist at least five times your body weight, for example, when you are jumping (see page 90).

### Progression
You can develop this exercise by using increasingly strong bands, by doubling your band or by tying the band around the back of a chair seat rather than holding the ends.

*Picking flowers* *There are many everyday tasks that require us to squat down on our haunches. When we stand up from this position, we use a powerful leg press.*

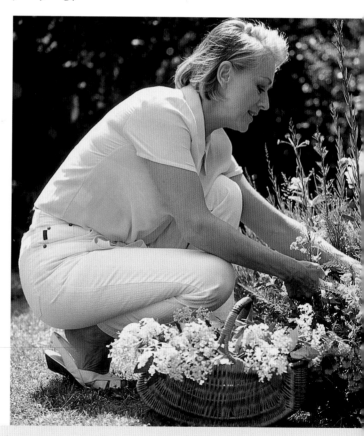

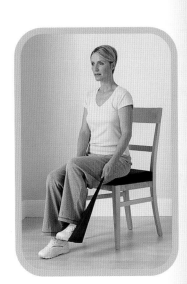

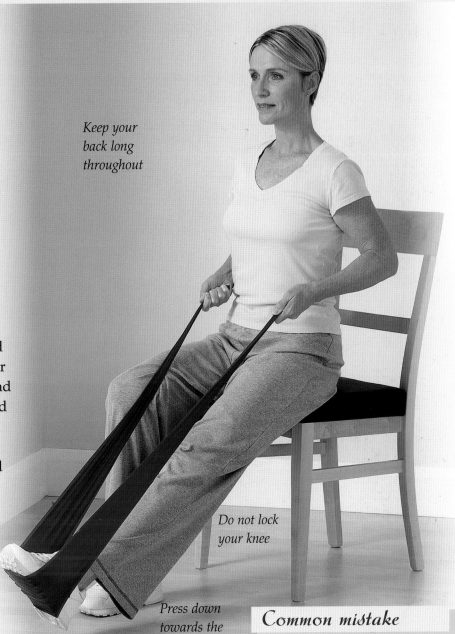

*Keep your back long throughout*

*Do not lock your knee*

*Press down towards the floor*

*Do not overflex your foot*

**1** Sit tall with your feet and legs hip-width apart and your knees directly over your ankles. Place a resistance band under the ball of one foot and hold one end firmly in each hand. Check your pelvic tilt, tighten your abdominals and lift your thigh toward your chest.

**2** Tighten the band by pulling your hands toward your hips. Keeping them steady, slowly press your foot against the band until your leg is straight. Count to 3 as you straighten, hold, count to 3 to release. Rest briefly and repeat. Move the band to the other leg, then repeat.

### Adaptation

*If you find holding the band taut uncomfortable, hold it against the chair seat instead.*

*Common mistake*

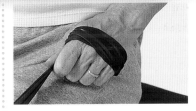

★ Do not wrap the band around your hand.

# LEG CURL

This exercise targets the large muscles at the back of the thigh (the hamstrings) which straighten the hip and bend the knees.

The hamstrings are potentially powerful muscles but they are often weaker than they should be when compared to their opposite muscle group: the quadriceps. The hamstrings are used in everyday activities such as stair-climbing and for many sports, but they need extra resistance to improve strength and load the bones. The Leg Curl loads bones effectively only when you use ankle weights.

## Progression

Master the exercise using a light ankle weight, then increase the weight and height of the lift to a limit of 8 cm (3 in). (The safety limit is 9 kg (20 lbs).)

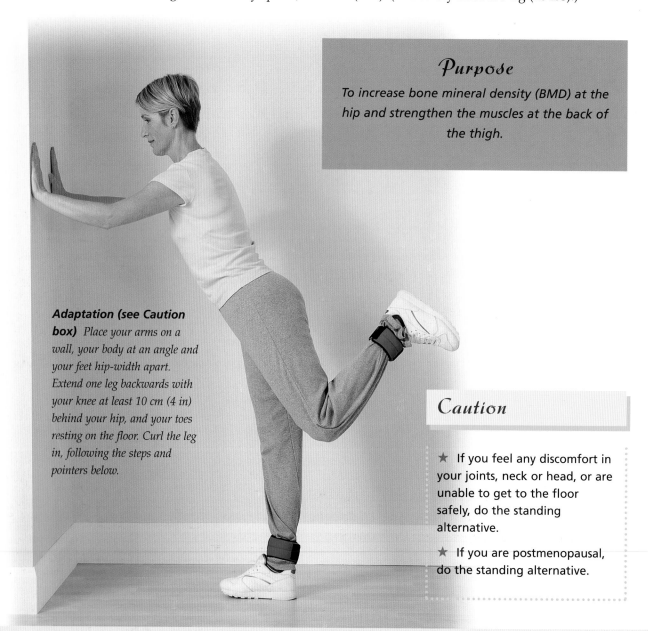

*Purpose*
To increase bone mineral density (BMD) at the hip and strengthen the muscles at the back of the thigh.

**Adaptation (see Caution box)** *Place your arms on a wall, your body at an angle and your feet hip-width apart. Extend one leg backwards with your knee at least 10 cm (4 in) behind your hip, and your toes resting on the floor. Curl the leg in, following the steps and pointers below.*

## Caution

★ If you feel any discomfort in your joints, neck or head, or are unable to get to the floor safely, do the standing alternative.

★ If you are postmenopausal, do the standing alternative.

**1** Kneel on all-fours with your legs hip-width apart. Your elbows should be bent under your shoulders, with your forearms and palms flat on the floor. Check your pelvic tilt, tighten your abdominals and slide one leg out behind you. Flex your foot and lift it about 3 cm. Lengthen your leg.

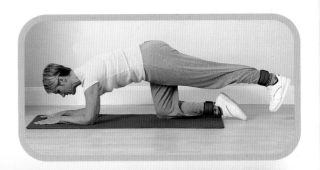

**2** Continue to lift your straight leg until your knee is just above the level of your hip, then curl the lower leg inwards to a count of 3 until your ankle is directly above your knee.

*Keep your heel in line with your knee and hip*

*Your foot should stay flexed*

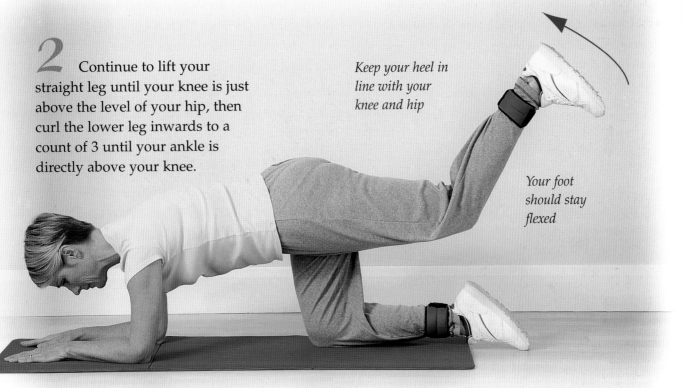

**3** Taking care not to overarch your back, lift your leg about 3 cm, hold, then lower with control for a count of 3. Rest, then repeat. Repeat with the other leg.

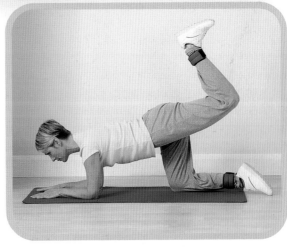

# STRAIGHT LEG LIFT

This exercise targets the quadriceps muscles of the thigh that cross both the front of the hip (the hip flexors) and the front of the knees (the knee extensors). They are powerful muscles that you use to some extent in all weight-bearing activities; and are the most important muscles for cycling or kicking. This exercise works the four quadriceps muscles and loads the hip. It is also excellent for reducing instability and discomfort arising from incorrect alignment of the knee joints. Keeping these muscles strong is important for independence as you grow older.

Performing this exercise in a controlled way and progressing step-by-step is very important if you are to get the maximum benefit from the work.

**Progression**
Add a weight when you have mastered the Straight Leg Lift. Progress further by lifting the heel about 10 cm (4 in) off the floor. Do not lift higher than your other thigh. Progress even further by increasing the weight.

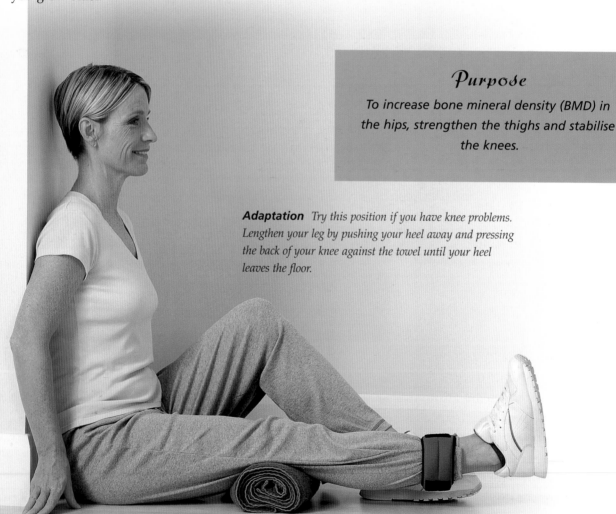

*Purpose*
To increase bone mineral density (BMD) in the hips, strengthen the thighs and stabilise the knees.

**Adaptation**  *Try this position if you have knee problems. Lengthen your leg by pushing your heel away and pressing the back of your knee against the towel until your heel leaves the floor.*

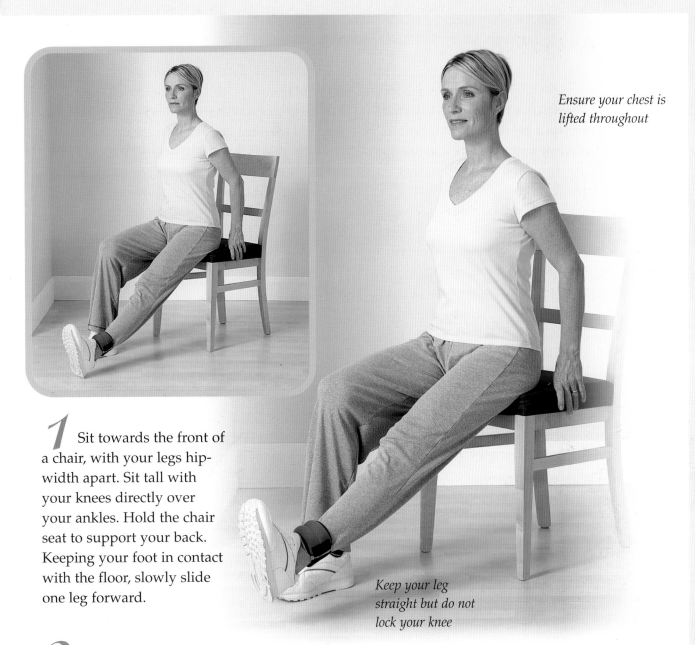

*Ensure your chest is lifted throughout*

*Keep your leg straight but do not lock your knee*

*1* Sit towards the front of a chair, with your legs hip-width apart. Sit tall with your knees directly over your ankles. Hold the chair seat to support your back. Keeping your foot in contact with the floor, slowly slide one leg forward.

*2* Lengthen your leg as much as possible by pushing your heel away, then check your pelvic tilt and tighten your abdominals and thigh muscles. Count to 3 as you lift your foot slowly, about 5 cm, hold, then lower it with control for 3. Rest, then repeat with the other leg.

## Caution

★ If you feel any pain or discomfort in your back or knees during this exercise, check your pelvic tilt, abdominals and leg alignment. If the problem persists, discontinue this exercise and seek advice from your doctor.

★ Avoid the temptation to lift too high or use ankle weights too soon.

# THIGH LIFT

This exercise targets several muscles that bend the hip joint, but the important one for bone loading is the psoas muscle which crosses from the femur to the lumbar spine. This exercise has been shown to be effective on its own, rather than as part of a package; it is usual to evaluate at least six weight-training exercises together. Performed at least three times a week using a 5 kg (11 lb) weight on the mid-thigh, this lift has been shown to maintain BMD in postmenopausal women.

You use these muscles a little when you lift your foot to step on to a bus and a lot when you lean backward if sitting without a support.

## Progression

Master the exercise using just the weight of your leg, then add a light weight around your thigh as shown and lift just 3 cm (1 in). Progress by lifting another 3 cm (1 in) without letting your chest or lower back sag. Progress further by moving the weight further down your thigh toward your knee, then increase the weight.

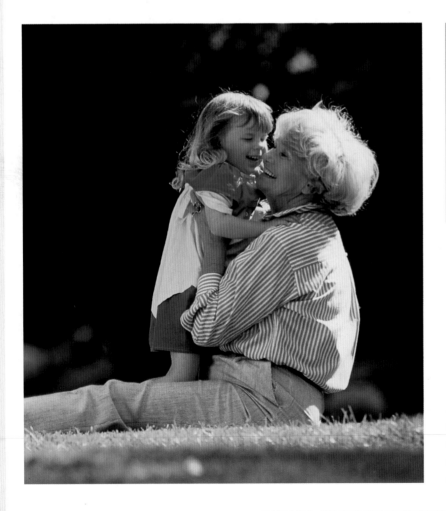

### Purpose
To increase bone mineral density (BMD) in the lower spine and strengthen the muscles at the front of the hips and thighs.

**Active living** *Even simple, everyday activities require strength; the woman in this position requires strong hip and thigh muscles to resist the weight of the child and her own upper body.*

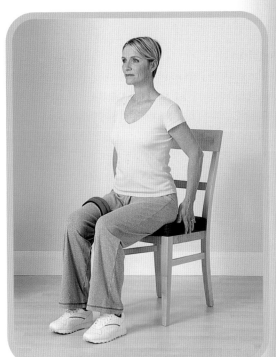

*Keep your chest lifted*

*Do not place the weight directly over or around your knee joint*

*Do not overarch your back*

1 Sit toward the front of a chair with your feet hip-width apart and your knees directly over your ankles. Secure a weight across the top of one thigh. Sit tall and hold the chair to support your back. Check your pelvic tilt and tighten your abdominals.

2 Tense the muscles of your weighted thigh as if to lift the leg. Press down against the floor with your supporting foot. Re-tighten your abdominals and lift your weighted thigh about 5 cm. Count to 3 as you lift, hold, count to 3 lower. Rest, then repeat with your other leg.

## Caution

★ If you feel any pain in your back, hip or knees, other than mild stiffness following this exercise, try it without weights. If the pain persists, seek advice from your doctor.

★ Do not lift your leg higher than shown.

# WRIST CURL

Most women have weak arms compared to their legs, so it is well worth doing some upper body exercises. The wrist is particularly vulnerable to osteoporotic fracture, so the next few exercises concentrate on increasing wrist BMD. The Wrist Curl targets the muscles which cross the wrist. To identify these muscles, hold your forearm gently in one hand while you clench your other hand into a fist; you will feel your muscles contracting. The muscles provide your grip power for twisting the lids off jars.

The wrist is an extremely flexible joint which allows the hand to move in all three planes like an anglepoise lamp. The forearm muscles pull on the wrist bones as you lift the weight, and the force is greater while you lower the weight because the muscles control the pull of gravity.

### Progression
Master the Wrist Curl exercise using a light weight, and progress further by increasing the weight. (The safety limit is 5 kg (11 lbs) in each hand.)

### *Purpose*
*To increase bone mineral density (BMD) in your wrists and to strengthen the muscles of the wrists and forearms.*

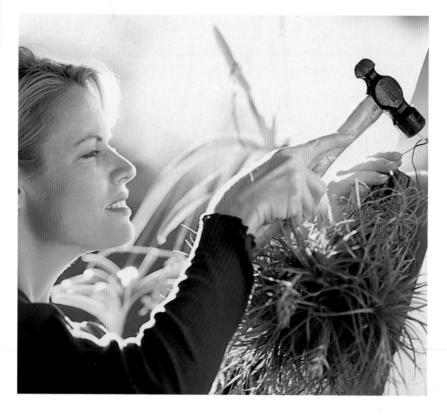

### Alternative
*Both these exercises can be performed double-handed provided you can find a suitable surface, such as a waist-height narrow table or bench, where your back can be erect and your forearms supported.*

**Loading the wrist bones**
*Hammering like this uses a wrist curl action with the wrist in a different position; the impact will probably help to load the wrist bones.*

## *Caution*

★ If you experience pain at the end of the upward or downward movement you have gone beyond your natural range.

*1* Sit toward the front of a chair with your feet hip-width apart and your knees over your ankles. Hold a dumb-bell in an underhand grip, with your wrist horizontal and in line with your elbow. Support your forearm with your other hand, resting it on your thigh. Lean forward slightly.

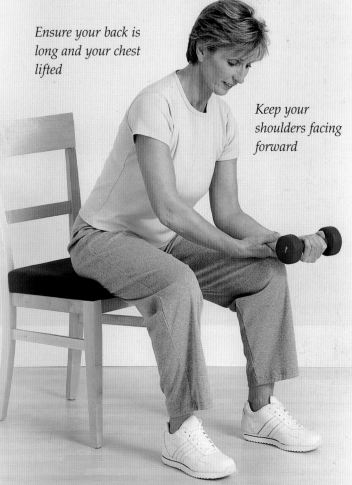

*Ensure your back is long and your chest lifted*

*Keep your shoulders facing forward*

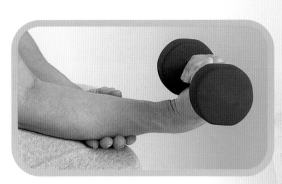

*2* Count to 3 to curl the dumb-bell upward, moving only your wrist. Hold.

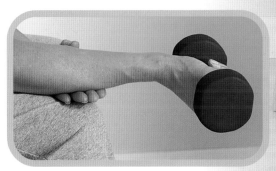

*3* Count to 3 to lower the weight until your wrist is fully extended downward, and return it the start position. Rest, then repeat. Repeat with your other arm.

*4* Turn your forearm over and repeat the exercise using an overhand grip.

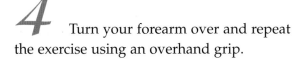

# ARM CURL

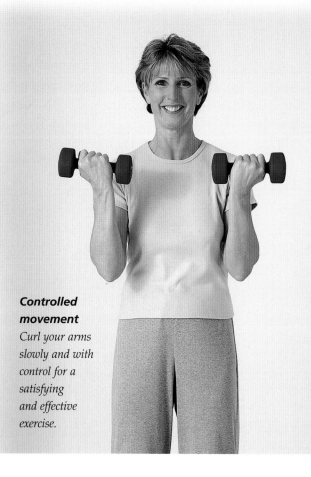

**Purpose**

*To increase the bone mineral density (BMD) in your wrists and to strengthen the muscles at the front of your arms.*

This exercise, often referred to as a biceps curl, targets the biceps muscle at the front of your upper arm – the muscle that everyone pinches to see if you are strong. It is attached to the radius and the humerus bones.

The exercise uses the biceps muscles to bend the elbow joints, and then allows them to straighten again resisting the force of gravity acting on the hand-held weights. These curls will make your biceps feel firm and give your arm a good line without becoming bulgy. You'll find it easier to manage heavy shopping bags as your muscles increase in strength. This exercise will help to improve BMD in the wrists, because they are also involved in the lift.

**Controlled movement**
*Curl your arms slowly and with control for a satisfying and effective exercise.*

## Progression

If you find this exercise hard, then try with one arm at a time. Master the technique with a light weight, then progress by increasing the weight. (The safety limit is 9 kg (20 lbs) in each hand.)

## Caution

★ The wrists should not move during this exercise. If you find it difficult to keep them fixed, use a lighter weight.

★ Do not lock the elbows at the end of the lowering movement and do not touch your shoulders on the lift.

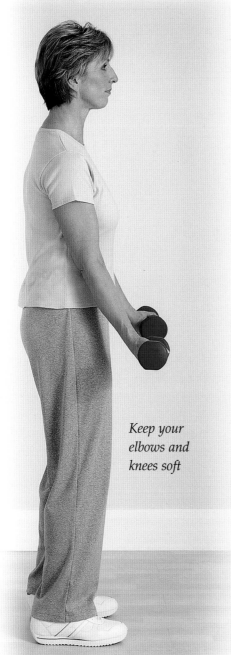

*Make sure that your wrists stay straight*

*Hold your upper body still*

*Keep your abdominals tight*

*Distribute your weight evenly between both feet and think tall*

*Keep your elbows and knees soft*

**2** Curl your arms upward toward your shoulders. Count to 3 as you lift, hold, and count to 3 to lower. Rest, then repeat.

**1** Stand tall with your feet hip-width apart and your knees bent slightly. Your arms should be a little more than shoulder-width apart. Hold the dumb-bells in an underhand grip with your palms facing forward. Check your pelvic tilt, tighten your abdominals, press your shoulders back and down, and lengthen your arms.

## Common mistake

★ Do not lean back as you lift your arms or swing the weight upward. Think of keeping the body firm and still as you lift and lower.

# ARM PRESS

> ## Purpose
> To increase the bone mineral density (BMD) in your wrists and to strengthen the muscles at the back of your arms and in your back.

This exercise targets the muscles across the chest and upper arm (pectorals) and at the back of your upper arm (triceps); it also involves your wrist muscles, particularly when the 'spring' is added to the press (see Progression). It is a vertical press-up, which is much easier to perform than a horizontal one. As well as being good for your wrist BMD, it helps you to maintain your upper body muscles and a good bust line. The triceps area, in particular, can become 'baggy' as you get older, if neglected. You need to hold your body firm in this exercise, which requires concentration. Think of your body as a rigid plank of wood, with your arms doing all the work.

## Progression

You can add impact by performing the spring alternative shown (*right*). Push away a little more powerfully until your hands leave the wall and then land carefully, rolling your weight through your fingers, palm and heel of your hand.

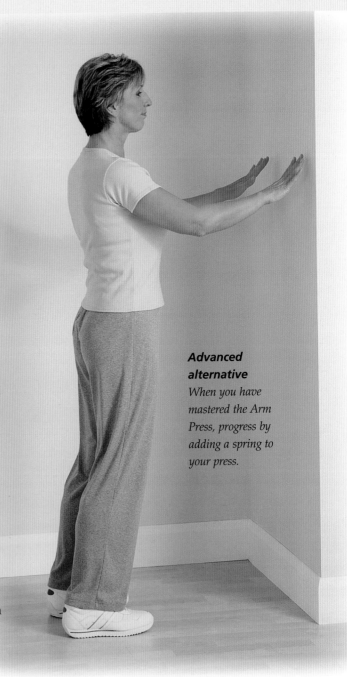

**Advanced alternative**
*When you have mastered the Arm Press, progress by adding a spring to your press.*

## Caution

★ If you have a shoulder injury, place your hands below shoulder height.

★ If you have arthritis in your fingers, shoulders or neck, do not perform the alternative above.

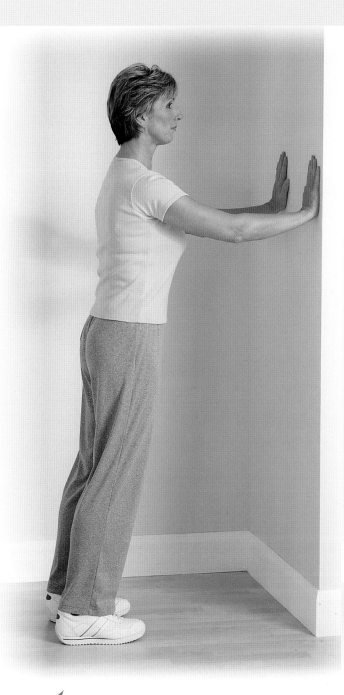

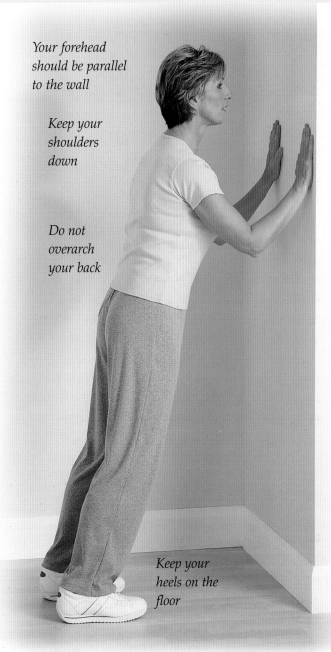

*Your forehead should be parallel to the wall*

*Keep your shoulders down*

*Do not overarch your back*

*Keep your heels on the floor*

*1* Stand facing a wall with your feet hip-width apart. Place your palms, fingers upward, on the wall at shoulder height. Your arms should be shoulder-width apart, and your elbows extended but not locked. Check your pelvic tilt and tighten your abdominals.

*2* Keeping your spine and neck long, bend your elbows and lower your body toward the wall. Press against the wall to return to your start position. Count to 3 as you lower, hold, count to 3 to return. Rest, then repeat.

# SHOULDER PRESS

## Purpose

*To increase the bone mineral density (BMD) in your wrists and to strengthen the muscles at the back of your arms and in your back.*

This exercise targets the muscles across the top of the shoulder joint and the triceps at the back of the arm; it requires a good range of movement in the shoulder. You use these muscles when you lift something on to a high shelf. The exercise also involves your pectoral muscles and the muscles of the upper back and spine, so it should help improve BMD in the spine. The spine has to be like a firm pole to keep the weight of the arms and dumb-bells in position. If you do not observe the caution box (below), the risk of shoulder injury is high.

## Progression

Start cautiously with a light weight and increase gradually as you become more competent (the safety limit is 7 kg (15 lbs) in each hand). For variety, turn your forearms and palms inward to perform the press. The seated version helps to stabilise the lower back and is therefore safer when using heavier weights. Do not perform the standing alternative unless you are very competent.

## Caution

★ Protect your back and shoulders by pushing directly upwards. Do not lean forwards or back; keep your arms just in front of your ears.

★ Don't worry if your shoulders click, as long as it is not painful.

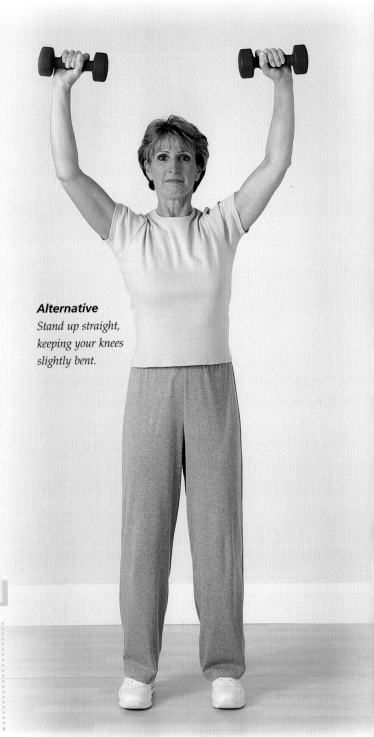

**Alternative**
*Stand up straight, keeping your knees slightly bent.*

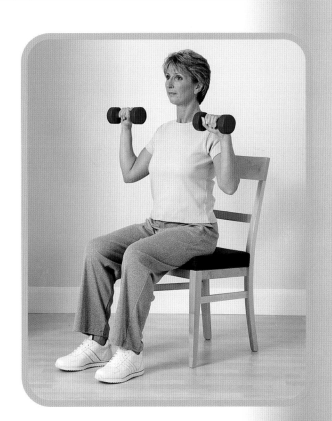

*Push directly
upward*

*Do not
lock your
elbows*

*Keep your
shoulders
down*

*Avoid
overarching
your back*

*1* Sit with your feet and legs hip-width apart. Hold the dumb-bells in a 'thumb under' grip with your elbows bent and your hands a little wider than shoulder-width apart. Your palms should face forward with your knuckles up toward the ceiling. Check your pelvic tilt and tighten your abdominals.

## Common mistake

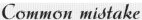

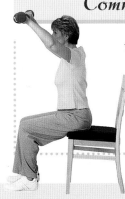

★ Don't push your arms forward: this places strain on your back.

★ Don't allow your arms to swing as you lift or lower.

*2* Press the dumb-bells directly up until your arms are as straight as possible but not locked. Count to 3 as you lift, hold, count to 3 as you lower to the start position. Rest, then repeat.

# CHEST PRESS

## Purpose

To increase BMD in your wrists and spine and strengthen the muscles of your chest, shoulders and back.

This exercise targets the muscles that straighten the forearm and many supporting muscles in the back and chest, including the pectorals. You use these muscles to push heavy objects around, for example, when you move furniture or push children on a swing. This exercise will firm up your bust line, as well as helping to improve BMD in the spine.

The arm action is similar to that in the Shoulder Press but the forces are acting in a different direction so the loading on the spine will be different. It is less demanding of the supporting muscles and is feasible even if you have a poor range of movement in the shoulder.

## Progression

Increase the weights to work your muscles harder. (The safety limit is 9 kg (20 lbs) in each hand.) This floor chest press effectively loads the wrists and spine. Benefits to the spine are greater if you go to a gym and use a chest press machine.

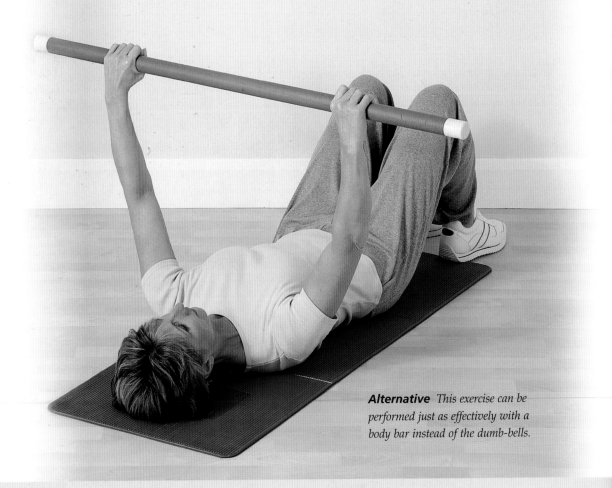

**Alternative** *This exercise can be performed just as effectively with a body bar instead of the dumb-bells.*

*1* Lie on a mat with your knees bent, your feet and legs hip-width apart and your feet on the floor. Hold the dumb-bells in an overhand grip, your palms facing forward, and your knuckles facing the ceiling. Your arms should be bent and slightly wider than shoulder-width apart. Check your pelvic tilt and tighten your abdominals. Press the dumb-bells upward, without locking the elbows, to reach the start position.

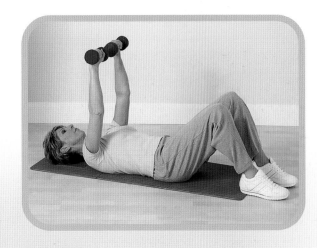

*Keep the dumb-bells in line with your chest, not your neck*

*Avoid overarching or flattening your back*

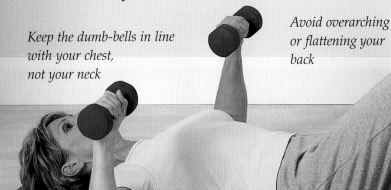

*2* Slowly lower the dumb-bells to a count of 3 by bending your elbows, allowing your arms to move out to the sides until they touch the floor. Rest, but maintain the arm and wrist position. Press the dumb-bells up again to a count of 3. Hold in the start position, then repeat.

## Caution

★ Attention to the position of the weight is particularly important for safety in this exercise.

★ If you experience dizziness when you get up from the floor, make sure you come up slowly.

## Alternative

*You can do an effective chest press while seated by using a band instead of dumb-bells if you are unable to get to the floor safely.*

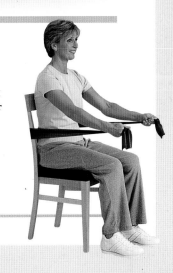

# ALL-FOURS

This exercise is a weight-bearing exercise for your arms rather than your legs. It targets many of the same muscles as the Arm Press (see page 68), particularly the pectorals, triceps and wrist flexors. The loading on your wrist, however, is greater than in an arm press. When you are on all-fours, your forearms are carrying nearly half of your body weight. By moving the position of your hands on the floor you can vary the direction of loading and the way that your wrist muscles are pulling to support your weight.

This exercise, along with the Arm Press and the Wrist Press, Twist & Pull (see page 76), forms a set of bone-loading exercises, which load the wrist in different directions. Research has shown that, when all these exercises were done three times a week by postmenopausal women, they improved BMD in the wrists by almost six per cent.

You load your wrist in a similar way when you polish a table, clean windows or push a child in a pushchair. Pushing a pushchair probably achieves just as much as this set of exercises, provided the child weighs over 9 kg (20 lbs). Going uphill with a pushchair provides a wrist press, downhill a wrist pull, and awkward kerbs provide a similar experience to the next exercise.

## Caution

★ If you experience any pain during this exercise, omit the forward movement, but spend time on all-fours. If the pain persists, stop.

★ If your wrists are painful as a result of this exercise, keep your body weight evenly distributed between your knees and hands.
If the pain persists, stop and do more Wrist Curls (see page 64).

*1* Kneel on all-fours with your wrists directly under your shoulders, your fingers facing forward, your knees and feet slightly apart and your knees above your hips. Check your pelvic tilt and tighten your abdominals. Move your body and hips slightly forward, so that most of your body weight is over your wrists.

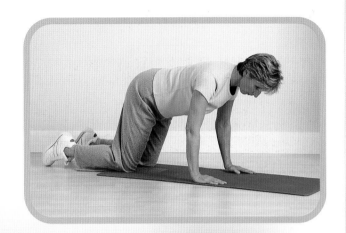

*Ensure the back of your neck is long and in line with your spine*

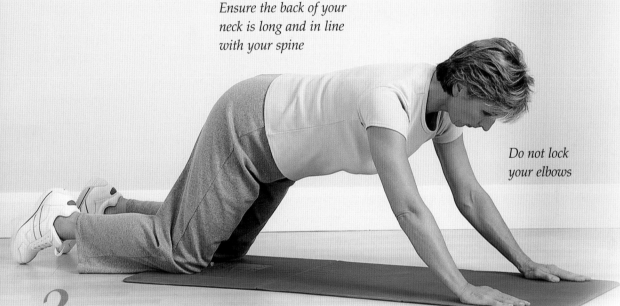

*Do not lock your elbows*

*2* Making small, controlled movements, walk your hands forward as far as you can without overarching your back or moving your knees or feet. Hold, then walk your hands back to the start position. Rest, then repeat.

*3* Walk your hands out to either side, as far as you can, keeping your body rigid. Hold, then walk your hands back to the start position. Rest, then repeat.

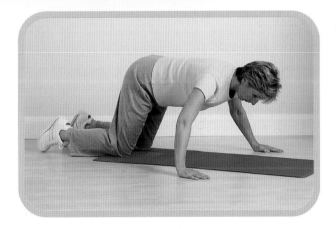

# WRIST PRESS, TWIST & PULL

These exercises target the muscles controlling the movement of your hands: the wrist flexors and extensors. These are the muscles you use to grip and twist bottle tops, wring wet towels and push a shopping trolley. They load your wrist bone in many directions. You'll need a partner, preferably of a similar size to yourself. If you have to rely on someone bigger, make sure they adjust their strength to meet yours. Use a smooth pole, at least 60 cm (2 ft) long, such as a body-bar or broom handle. If you cannot find a pole, you could do some arm wrestling at the kitchen table.

There are three exercises here: the press, the twist and the pull. In each exercise, your partner will be working against you, thus generating high resistant forces. You should feel these forces all the way down your body, proving how many muscle groups are being challenged.

## Progression

Generate as much force as you can, counting to three as you press, twist or pull. Hold for a second before you release your effort.

**Alternative** *If you do not have a partner to work with, you can do the Wrist Twist by using a pole or broom on your own as if you were wringing out a towel.*

## Purpose

To increase bone mineral density (BMD) in the wrists. It also strengthens muscles in the trunk, shoulders and forearms.

## Caution

★ Avoid being competitive, keep the pole equidistant between both partners.

★ If you have arthritis in your hands, do not do this exercise.

*1* **Start** Stand opposite your partner with your feet slightly wider than hip-width apart and your knees bent. Hold the bar with both hands shoulder-width apart, one hand using an underhand grip, the other overhand. Check your pelvic tilt and tighten your abdominals.

*2* **Press** Push upward with your underhand palm and downward with the other as if trying to rotate the ends of the pole. Your partner should press in the opposite direction. Change your grips around and repeat in the opposite direction. Rest, then repeat.

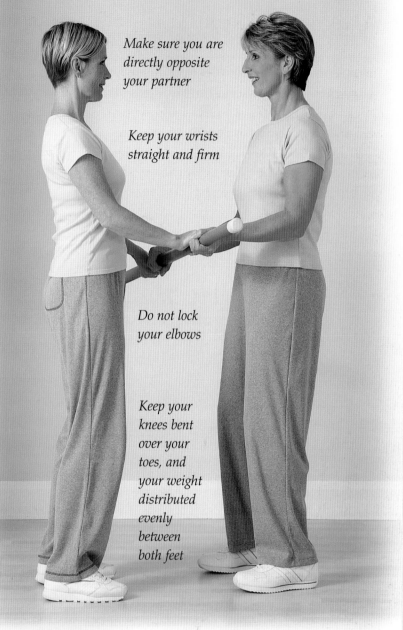

*Make sure you are directly opposite your partner*

*Keep your wrists straight and firm*

*Do not lock your elbows*

*Keep your knees bent over your toes, and your weight distributed evenly between both feet*

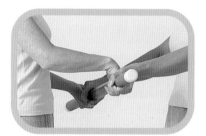

*3* **Twist** Return to your start position. Twist the pole, as if wringing a towel. Your partner should twist in the opposite direction. Change your grips and repeat the exercise in the opposite direction. Rest, then repeat.

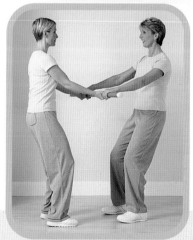

*4* **Pull** Return to your start position. Hold the pole with an underhand grip, while your partner uses an overhand grip. Pull in toward your waist as your partner pulls in the opposite direction. Reverse your grip and repeat. Rest, then repeat.

# ABDOMINAL LIFT

This exercise targets the muscles that form the front wall of your lower abdomen. These are important muscles as they support your trunk and, indirectly, your back and spine. They need to be strong to perform your bone-loading exercises effectively; all the forces generated by your arms and legs are supported by the centre of your body. These muscles are important for maintaining good posture and correct pelvic tilt. Strong abdominals also give you a trim figure and reduce your risk of falls. Slack abdominal muscles allow your middle to bulge outward and can lead to back pain. Focus on tightening the triangle of muscles spreading from your waistline to your pubic bone.

## Purpose

*To strengthen the abdominals. This will ensure good support for the back, safe exercising and improved posture.*

## Unsafe exercise

★ Out-dated sit-ups should be avoided because they increase the risk of vertebral fracture.

**Advanced alternative**  *When you have mastered the Abdominal Lift shown opposite, try this position for an extra challenge.*

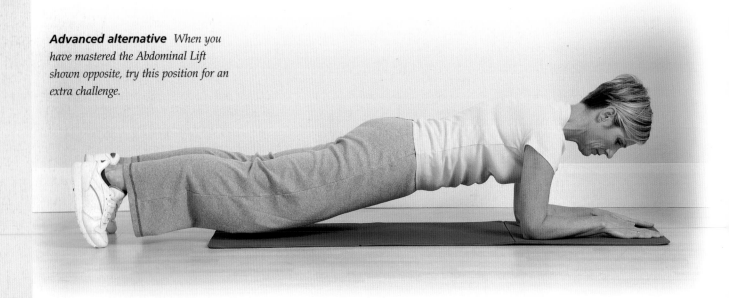

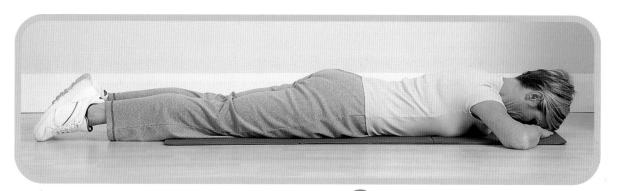

**1** Lie face-down with your forehead on your folded hands. Position your legs about 5 cm apart. Check your pelvic tilt.

**2** Breathe in, then breathe out as you contract your abdominals and lift your navel in toward your spine. Hold, then release back to the start. Rest, then repeat.

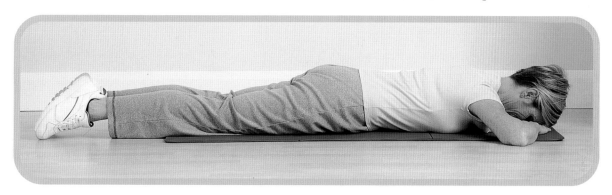

**3** Progress by positioning your arms, elbows and shoulders as shown. Lift your navel, abdominals and hips off the floor. Try not to over-tilt your pelvis. Breathe out as you contract, lift and pull in. Hold, and breathe in as you release. Rest, then repeat.

*Keep the back of your neck long and your shoulders down*

*Relax your buttock muscles*

*Maintain your pelvic tilt and keep tightening your abdominals*

# Flexibilty Stretches

## Purpose

*Over time, these stretches will improve your suppleness and reduce the risk of injury in both everyday and recreational activities.*

A cool-down using flexibility stretches, gentle relaxation and brief revitalising circulation exercises is an essential finish to every exercise programme. The exercises have left your muscles warm and pliant, so this is a good time to develop your joint flexibility. Begin by repeating the warm-up stretches (see pages 32–7); the emphasis now should be on developing each of these stretches as far as you can, comfortably.

Add the two stretches shown here to provide more supported positions for your hamstring and inner thigh muscles. These muscles are important to stretch and they respond particularly well to longer, developmental stretches. Extend the duration of the stretches gradually from ten seconds each to one minute each.

## Effective stretching

★ Put on an extra top to retain body heat and to feel more comfortable.

★ It is important to do these longer stretches gradually.

★ Move slowly with control to take your muscles into the fully stretched positions shown.

★ Hold until you feel the tightness subside.

★ Then, on an out-breath, move gently further into the stretch. Try to relax into the stretch.

★ Release any tension in the rest of the body, especially the shoulders.

★ To finish, move slowly out of the stretch again.

## Relax and revitalise

★ Spend a few minutes relaxing.

★ Lie on your back on the floor, with knees raised slightly.

★ Tense and relax your muscles to feel the difference in your face, shoulders, hands, all the way down.

★ Do a full body stretch to wake you up again.

★ Revitalise by doing the circulation exercises on page 26.

## Caution

★ Never bounce in a stretch. This can tighten the muscle you are trying to stretch, and may cause injury.

★ Remain seated a few moments after the lying stretch. Get up slowly to avoid dizziness.

## Unsafe exercise

★ Do not touch your toes with straight legs to stretch the back and hamstrings. This outdated stretch carries an increased risk of both back and eye injuries.

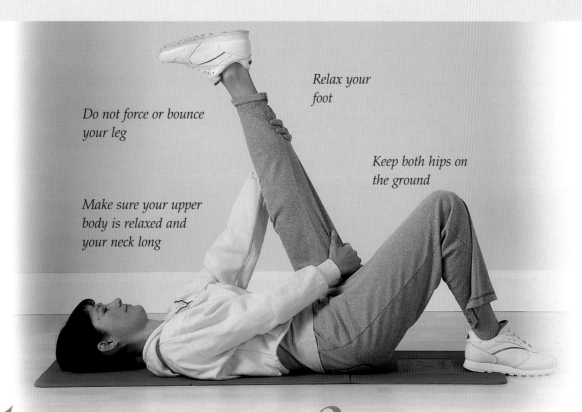

*Do not force or bounce your leg*

*Relax your foot*

*Keep both hips on the ground*

*Make sure your upper body is relaxed and your neck long*

*1* **Hamstring stretch** Lie on your back with both knees bent and your feet flat on the floor. Check your pelvic tilt, tighten your abdominals and, keeping the knee bent, lift one leg in toward your chest. Take hold of the back of your thigh with both hands. Relax for a count of 10.

*2* Slowly straighten your leg until you feel a stretch in the back of your raised thigh. Slide your outside hand up on to the lower leg so your whole leg is supported. If you feel the stretch subside, bring the leg gently a little further toward your chest. Hold for a count of 10 or more. Relax, then return to the start and repeat on the other leg.

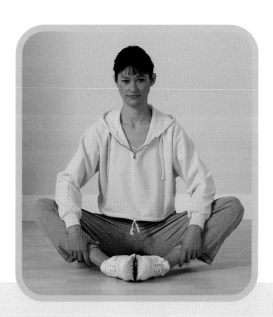

*1* **Inner thigh stretch** Sit on a folded mat with the soles of your feet together, your back long and your chest lifted. Place your arms on your legs as shown, and allow your knees to open naturally. Check your pelvic tilt and tighten your abdominals.

*2* Use your forearms and then your hands to press your legs down gently, until you feel a stretch along your inner thighs. If you feel the stretch subside, lean forward slightly for a deeper stretch. Hold for a count of 10 or more.

# ACTIVITIES FOR LIFE

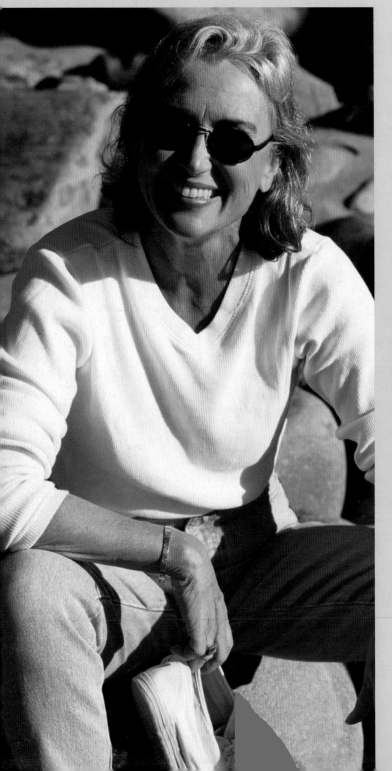

This section contains physical activities for increasing bone strength that you can include in your daily life, both inside and outside of the home. They are weight-bearing activities, which means that you are on your legs and your skeleton is supporting the weight of your body. While these exercises are beneficial for your hips and spine, they won't benefit your wrist bones. Weight-bearing is not the same as weight-training, which is about lifting weights to increase muscle and bone strength.

The exercises in this chapter are arranged in order of increasing intensity. If you have not been exercising regularly before now, start by introducing some gentle activities into your life such as those on pages 83–9. If you are young, healthy and already lead an active life, the higher-impact exercises on pages 90–93 will improve your bone strength.

## WALKING

If you are not in the habit of taking any exercise at all, then a brief daily walk outside the home is a good start. Most people achieve this every day without thinking of it as exercise, but if you are a person who drives everywhere in the car, it is worth adding up how much walking you have done in the last few days.

Women who walk more than 1.5 km (1 mile) a week (about three minutes of walking a day, on average), have a significantly higher BMD than those who walk less than that. Walking for longer periods makes no further difference to BMD, although it has many other health benefits. Other research has shown that women who habitually walk briskly have better BMD than those who tend to walk at a slower rate. It is better, therefore, to take regular short walks than long ones, and to concentrate on walking faster.

Hiking is great exercise and is likely to be good for your BMD and balance. The changing gradients and surfaces give a variety of stimulation for bones. As yet, however, there have been no formal studies on the benefits.

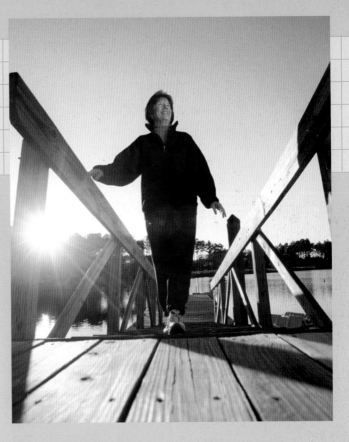

***Setting the pace*** *With the help of a car mileometer or an accurate map, plan out a 400 m (quarter of a mile) walk near your home or work. If you can walk the distance in five minutes, you are walking at a moderate pace. Aim to improve your time, and try to maintain this pace when walking elsewhere.*

## Getting started

★ Go for a brisk walk – at least five minutes long – every day.

★ Once you are warmed up, introduce some short spurts of a faster pace for a few seconds, reverting to your chosen speed in between. You should be breathing more than normal, but not breathless.

★ Walking for more than 10 minutes every day does not improve bone health any further, but walk–jog does, so if you can, follow the walk–jog programme instead (see pages 84–7).

★ Walking for half an hour once a week is not the same as five minutes daily. Little and often is the way to better bones.

# STAIR CLIMBING

If you live in a house with stairs you will be giving your leg muscles and skeleton a good daily workout without even realising it. Climbing stairs is an easy way to increase your daily activity level, and seems to be associated with good BMD and a low risk of fracture. Whenever possible, take the stairs instead of the escalator in a department store or public building, and instead of the lift in your work place or block of flats. If you live or work in a high-rise block, get out of the lift a storey earlier and walk the rest of the way.

You should aim to climb ten flights of ten stairs per day. If you live in a home with stairs, you will meet this target without thinking about it. But if you live in a bungalow or flat, then try to take the stairs whenever you are out and about.

## Caution

★ If you have osteoarthritis in your joints or problems with your knees or hips, then stair climbing is not the best exercise for you. Other forms of physical activity such as swimming would be better.

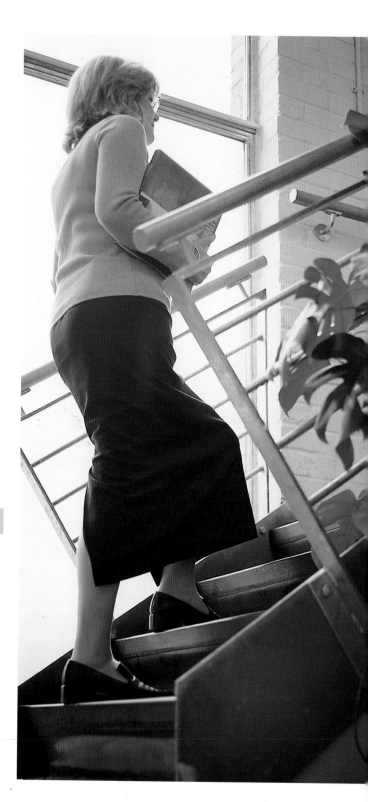

***Climb some stairs everyday*** *This is very good for your bones and the muscle power in your legs. Take the stairs instead of the lift whenever possible.*

# AQUAEROBICS

Exercise classes that take place in water, such as aquaerobics, use the resistance of the water to develop endurance, muscle strength, flexibility and balance. Any exercise that improves balance is important for reducing the risk of falls; it is especially helpful for people who have suffered a fall already and are fearful of falling again. You can work your body hard in the pool without risk, because you are cushioned by the water.

**Swimming pool exercise class**  *This is more fun than swimming lengths, and is very good for improving strength, flexibility and balance.*

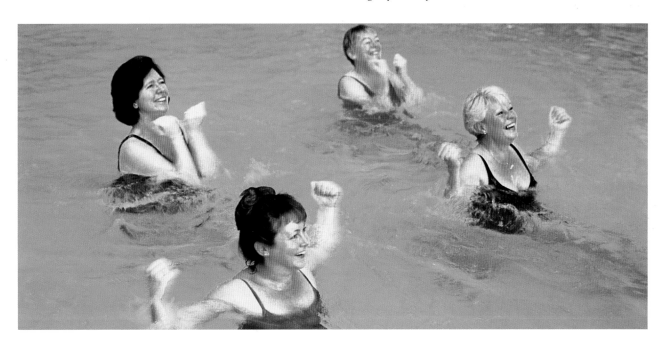

# T'AI CHI CH'UAN

Also known as 'T'ai Chi', this ancient practice is an excellent way to develop good balance and strong legs. It also instils a feeling of calmness, peace of mind and stability. It can be practised by people of all ages and is a confidence-booster for those who have suffered a fall.

T'ai Chi originated in China nearly 2000 years BC. It embraces a whole philosophy of life which has its roots in martial arts. It is also a meditative form of weight-bearing exercise which has been adapted to meet the demands and pace of modern life in the West. Balance, power and energy are the fundamental principles behind T'ai Chi.

It takes a long time to learn T'ai Chi properly and you need to join a class to do so. Once learned, however, it can be practised independently.

# WALK–JOG

### Purpose

This programme of alternate walking and jogging improves BMD in the spine and hips. It is also very good for cardiovascular health.

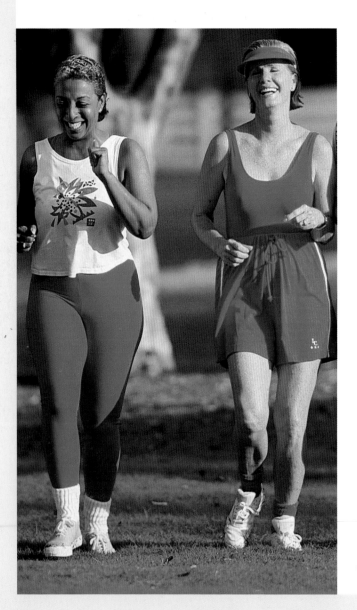

*A walk–jog* This activity can be started gently and built up gradually into a useful bone-loading exercise. It is suitable for those unaccustomed to regular exercise.

This is brisk walking interspersed with a bit of jogging (not to be confused with running, which is much more energetic). It used to be called 'Scout's pace' and it is a very efficient way of getting somewhere quickly without getting too hot, tired or breathless. Walk–jog can start as a bouncy walk and get more energetic as you improve.

This walk–jog programme has been proven to increase BMD in the spine and hips. It needs to be done three times a week in order to be effective, unless you already do other exercise. It should be done on non-consecutive days. Each session should last for about 20 minutes. It doesn't matter where you exercise; it could be in the park, while walking to the post box or to work. Wear sensible shoes and comfortable clothes and observe the 'Getting started' guidelines on pages 20 and 90.

### Caution

★ Do not jog if the ground is icy, nor if the weather is extremely cold or hot.

★ If you have asthma or are at risk from heart disease or falls, start with a regular walking programme for 12 weeks. Make sure you do not get breathless.

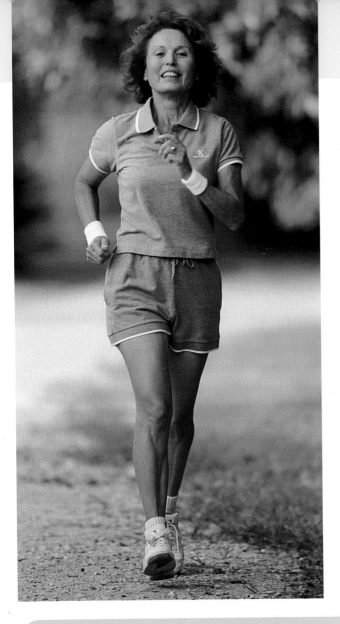

## Progression

If you are not used to exercise, start with Stage 1 below. If you are already a frequent brisk walker, start at Stage 2. If you already go jogging or running on a regular basis, consider some weight-training (see page 88).

### Caution

★ If you have arthritis, any leg or back pain, or a diagnosis of osteoporosis, then do not jog. Stick to a daily brisk short walk.

★ If you experience pain of any sort, slow down or stop.

| Stage 1 | Stage 2 | Stage 3 | Stage 4 |
|---------|---------|---------|---------|
| months 1–2 | months 3–4 | months 5–6 | month 7 onward |
| ★ Brisk walking only, for about 20 minutes<br><br>★ Try to increase your speed each day<br><br>★ Follow the same route and time yourself<br><br>★ Keep a record in your diary | ★ Introduce 6 jogging steps after every 60 walking steps<br><br>★ If you get hot or breathless, go back to walking for a few minutes, before starting again | ★ Increase your ratio of jogging to walking until you are doing about half and half, say walking for about half a minute, and jogging for half a minute | ★ Increase your ratio of jogging to walking until you are walking for half a minute and jogging for a whole minute<br><br>★ If you get too hot or breathless, do a bit more walking and a bit less jogging |

# WEIGHT-TRAINING

This is widely practised in gyms, sports clubs and health clubs. In these settings weight-training is done using free weights as in the home exercises and also using special weight-training machines. These machines contain stacks of weights that you raise and lower with your arms or legs using pulleys. Women of all ages do weight-training; you do not have to be strong.

An advantage of using weight-training machines in a gym environment is that there are different machines that allow you to exercise all the major muscle groups in the body. The machines are safe because your back is supported, the start position can be adjusted to suit you and the weights are within a cage so they cannot do any damage if you let them go.

Weight-training is often confused with weight-lifting which is a competitive sport in which very heavy weights are lifted, and bulging muscles are developed. It has nothing to do with the particular kind of training recommended in this book; muscles can get much stronger without becoming bulky.

Weight-training can be practised using small weights and many lifts; this is good for endurance but it does not improve BMD. To improve BMD you need to lift heavier weights quite slowly, a few times. It is important to work up to the heavier weights over several months so you do not injure yourself. Injuries, if they occur, are usually the result of 'too much, too soon' or poor technique.

If you have never done any weight-training, seek advice from a qualified instructor about technique and about how the machines work. Most gyms have free introductory sessions, so you can look until you find a gym that suits you. For improvements, train three times a week.

## Devise a gym programme

Explain to the gym instructor that you are working to improve your BMD. Ask for a programme that includes the following lifts:

**Lower body**

★ hip extension

★ hip flexion

★ hip adduction

★ hip abduction

★ leg extension

★ leg press

**Upper body**

★ lateral pull down

★ bench press

★ bicep curl

★ back extension

## Good technique

★ It is essential to start with light weights that you can lift easily until you have mastered the technique.

★ Make sure that your position is comfortable. Your back should be supported and your posture should be correct throughout.

★ Lift and lower the weight slowly. Count to three as you lift, and to three as you lower. Rest briefly before the next lift.

★ Breathe evenly throughout while counting out loud. You should not get breathless at any time.

★ Aim for eight lifts, resting for a second between each.

★ Aim to repeat your set of eight lifts twice more, resting for a minute between each set.

★ Remember to warm up first and stretch afterwards.

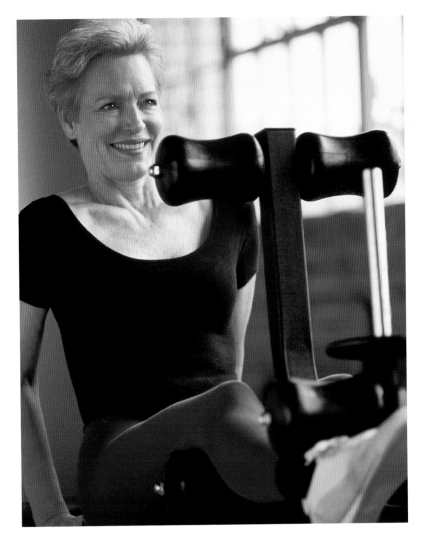

***Go to the gym*** *When you have mastered the exercises contained in this book, you can take your programme further by using weight machines in a gym. This woman is doing a leg extension.*

## Caution

★ Every woman is different, so it is important that you use a weight that is right for you. Follow the 1RM rule (see Progression). If in doubt about the most suitable weight to use, seek advice from a qualified instructor.

## Progression

When you have practiced correct lifting using a weight-training machine at least three times a week for one month, measure your 'one repetition maximum' (1RM). Lift a succession of weights once each, resting in between lifts. Increase the weight until you can no longer lift it once with acceptable form. This means smoothly and steadily through the movement, without any wobbles. The heaviest weight you can lift once is your 1RM. To train effectively for improving BMD, choose weights which are at least 70 per cent of your 1RM and do up to eight repetitions. If you can do more, then you need to use a heavier weight. As you improve and can complete eight repetitions easily, use a heavier weight. You should feel that the last lift of the last set is as much as you can manage.

# JUMPING

The exercises on the next four pages improve your BMD because of the impacts involved when your feet hit the ground but they carry a far higher risk of injury than the exercises contained in the main programme. Provided they are not practised to excess, they are recommended for healthy, premenopausal women.

Jumping is an energetic form of exercise, but it only takes a few minutes and you do not have to do many jumps to benefit your bones. It improves BMD in the hips (but not the spine) in premenopausal women, but unfortunately has no effect in postmenopausal women, even if they are taking HRT. Jumping also increases the power in your thighs and calves and improves your balance.

## Caution

★ Jumping is not recommended for women (even premenopausal women) who have poor balance, a history of falls or osteoarthritis in the back, legs or hips, or a history of joint pain.

## Getting Started

★ You will need to wear supportive shoes with cushioned, flexible shoes (e.g. trainers) to avoid joint injury. You will get warm, so wear comfortable, cotton clothes and drink water before and afterward.

★ Warm up following the exercises on pages 24–37. It is very important that you feel warm, loose and relaxed before you start this exercise.

## Variation

*If you prefer, try skipping. This activity is also good for shoulder flexibility and balance.*

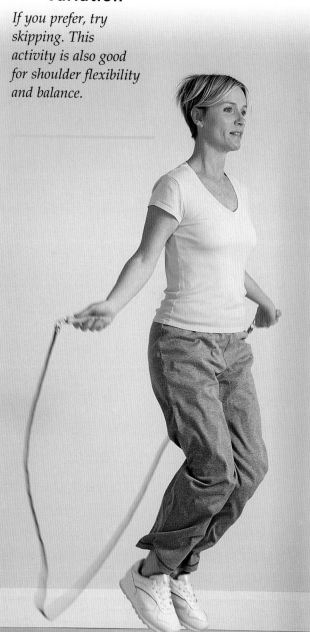

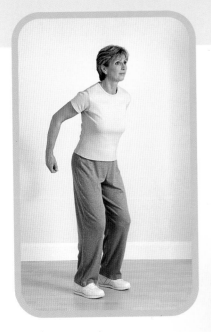

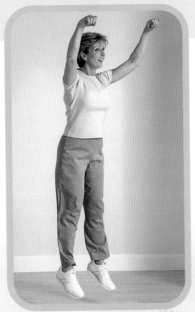

**2** Swing your arms forward, and jump into the air with both feet. Aim to jump about 8 cm (3 in) high – no more. The jump should be done in one smooth, quick movement.

**1** Find a well-ventilated space with a firm floor. Stand tall with your feet hip-width apart. Adjust your pelvic tilt and let your ankles, knees and hips give slightly. Bend your knees and swing your arms back to start.

**3** Bend your knees as you land. Repeat according to the programme below left.

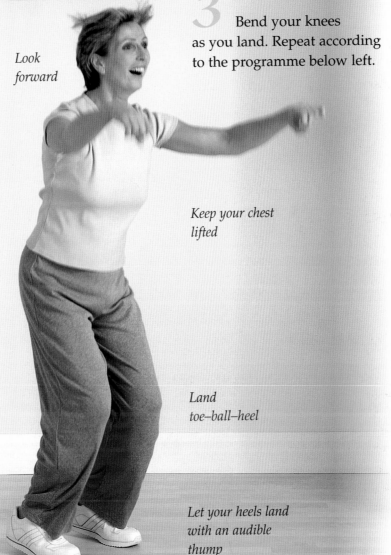

*Look forward*

*Keep your chest lifted*

*Land toe–ball–heel*

*Let your heels land with an audible thump*

### Progression

★ **Day 1** Start with a few experimental jumps

★ **Day 2** 5 jumps

★ **Day 3** 10 jumps

★ **Day 4** 20 jumps

★ **Day 5** 30 jumps

★ **Day 6** 50 jumps

★ **Day 7** Rest

NOTE: When doing 20 or more jumps, rest between each block of 10 by doing gentle stepping movements.

# CLASSES

Check your local community for exercise to music classes. They come in many forms and contain a variety of exercises. This variety is useful for bones as it loads the skeleton in lots of different ways. Aerobics classes and circuit-training include weight-bearing exercises and the best of these include both high- and low-impact work.

It is important to go to the class regularly, three times a week, unless you plan to include other forms of bone-loading activities in your weekly routine.

# DANCING

Since jumping and jogging are both good bone-loaders, it is likely that any dance that involves ground impact will have the same effect. Tap, Scottish and Irish dancing should all be effective.

Gentler forms of dance such as line dancing or ballroom dancing are very good for maintaining or improving balance, but they are unlikely to stimulate your bones.

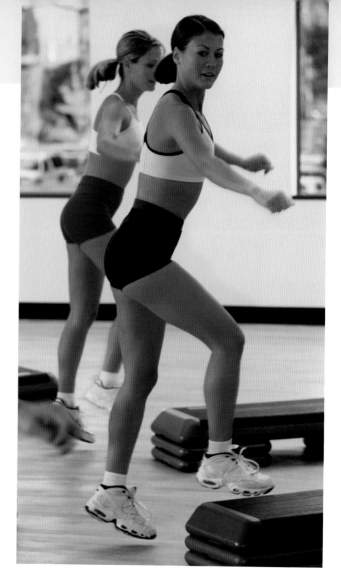

**Power step**  *This is a vigorous exercise that adds some jumping to stair climbing, so it is likely to load the hips and spine.*

## Caution

★ High-impact exercises carry a relatively high risk of injury. They are recommended only for premenopausal women.

## Active sports

Any sport that involves impact is likely to benefit your bones. Racquet sports such as tennis or squash should be effective, as will any sport that involves running and jumping, such as basketball.

Swimming and cycling, although very good for your health in other ways, are not effective for improving BMD.

# RUNNING

There is good evidence from studies in the USA that running stimulates BMD at both the spine and the hip in young women aged 20 years.

The usual recommendation is to run for 20–30 minutes, three times a week. This works well for reducing the risk of coronary heart disease and related problems. But there is evidence that shorter periods of running might do your skeleton just as much good.

In 20 minutes of running or jogging, your leading foot hits the ground at least 2000 times. However, fewer impacts are known to be effective for bone, so you may prefer to opt for intermittent jogging instead (see page 86).

Asphalt or grass are better running surfaces for your joints than tarmac. Wear light-coloured clothes if you go running in traffic, for safety.

## Caution

★ Jogging or running for long periods on hard surfaces increases the risk of osteoarthritis and should be avoided if you are vulnerable to this disease.

★ You will need to wear supportive shoes with cushioned, flexible shoes (e.g. trainers) to avoid joint injury. You will get warm, so wear comfortable, cotton clothes, and drink water before and afterward.

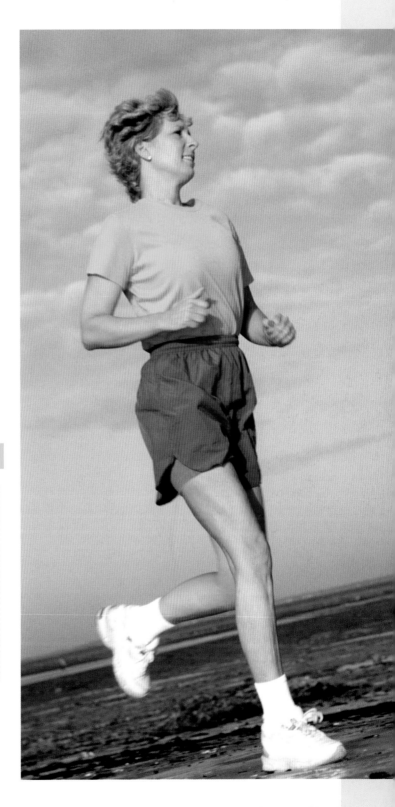

**Go for a run** *It will load your skeleton and it only needs a short run to be effective.*

# HEALTH QUESTIONNAIRE

| Ask yourself the following questions | If your answer is YES |
|---|---|
| ★ Have you been in hospital in the last six months?<br>★ Have you had any major illness or surgery in the last six months?<br>★ Do you have any current health problems for which you are under active treatment with medication, radiation or surgery?<br>★ Have you had a blackout or fallen more than twice in the past year? | Consult with your doctor about starting this new exercise program. Take the book with you to show him what you want to do. |
| ★ Do you have asthma or heart disease?<br>★ Do you get pain in your chest, neck or arm when exercising which does not go away when you rest for a few minutes? | Use your prescribed medication and avoid getting breathless, and avoid jumping or jogging unless you are used to doing this. |
| ★ Do you have high blood pressure or are you on treatment for it? | Limit any lift or muscle effort to five seconds. |
| ★ Do you have an artificial hip? | Look for special advice in caution boxes. |
| ★ Do you have tendonitis, bursitis or rheumatoid arthritis? | Avoid exercises which involve affected parts of your body. |
| ★ Do you have any abnormalities or pain when you walk such as a limp, painful joints or bunions?<br>★ Do you have chronic pain in your knees? | Avoid jogging or jumping and use seated alternatives of the home exercises. |
| ★ Do you have chronic pain in your hips or back?<br>★ Have you been diagnosed as osteoporotic (see page 95)?<br>★ Have you fallen once or twice in the past year?<br>★ Do you have poor balance or poor coordination? | Avoid jogging or jumping; use seated alternatives of the home exercises; limit weights to 4.5 kg (10 lbs); avoid the Shoulder Press exercise; and prioritise the Back Lift, Shoulder Mobiliser, Chest Stretch and balance exercises |

# HEALTH PROBLEMS AND EXERCISE

If you can answer 'no' honestly to all the questions, then all the home exercises should be safe for you, but if you are in any doubt, consult your doctor. If you have answered 'yes' to any question, follow the advice in the right-hand column and observe caution boxes.

## Osteoporosis

The diagnosis of osteoporosis is usually made when a bone scan using dual-energy X-ray absorptiometry (DXA) results in a 'T score' of 2.5 or more below normal values, when a bone fracture occurs with minimal impact (low trauma), or there are several risk factors (see page 11). Diagnoses based on Ultrasound need to be confirmed with DXA. A diagnosis of 'osteopenia', means you have a lower than normal BMD but you are not osteoporotic.

The exercises in this book are designed to reduce the risk of developing osteoporosis but if you already have this problem the exercise prescription must be modified. For example, high impact exercise is more likely to harm than help because it could cause a fracture. You need to concentrate on the good practice section and the balance exercises in order to protect you against falls, and the home exercises for your back in order to strengthen the supporting muscles round your spine and to help you to keep your spine straight.

## Osteoarthritis

This disease is often confused with osteoporosis because the names are similar; it is a disease of the joints, not the bones, from which many women suffer in later life.

The symptoms are pain at night and stiffness in the morning, typically affecting the hands, knees and hips. Impact loads must be avoided and exercise which is free of joint loading, such as swimming, is most beneficial.

The gentle options of the home exercises will maintain muscle strength around the joint and help to control pain, and stretching is useful for improving joint function and range of movement.

## Cardiovascular problems

Heart disease is common in later life but the home exercises are not designed to cause breathlessness, high pulse rates or raised blood pressure. If you do the gentle options slowly, with rests as prescribed on page 39, and pay attention to the cautions with each exercise, you should experience no cardio-respiratory distress.

## Falls

These are also common in later life and are the main cause of fractures, so if you have a history of falls avoid exercises which put you at risk. The good practice, balance and home exercises should safely improve your postural control.

# PHYSICAL ACTIVITY CHECKLIST

These questions are to help you check out both your present activity levels, and what you are currently able to do. Answering them honestly will enable you to identify those areas needing improvement and to tailor an exercise programme which is relevant for you. Find out how to test yourself safely by looking up the page numbers listed.

## Did you..?

| | Score |
|---|---|
| ★ Yesterday did you walk anywhere... | |
| at a brisk pace? | 3 |
| at a normal pace? | 1 |
| at a slow pace? | 0 |
| ★ Yesterday, did you walk for over 5 minutes? | 3 |
| ★ Yesterday, did you climb 5 flights of stairs? | 4 |
| ★ During the last week did you . . . | |
| go to a gym? | 5 |
| attend an exercise class? | 5 |
| play any other sport? | 5 |
| take any other exercise? | 5 |

Only score here if your activities were bone-loading (see Activities for life page 82)

Note your score and chart your improvements

DATE          TOTAL SCORE =

## Can you..?

| | Score |
|---|---|
| ★ Can you balance on one leg for 30 seconds? (see page 40) | 5 |
| ★ Can you reach the back of your neck? (see page 36) | 5 |
| ★ Can you walk on your toes for 20 steps? (see page 44) | 5 |
| ★ Can you walk for 5 minutes at 4 mph? (see page 83) | 5 |
| ★ Can you jog for 5 minutes at 5 mph? (see page 86) | 10 |
| ★ Can you raise your head 10 cm (4 in) off the floor in a back lift? (see page 46) | 5 |
| ★ Can you do 16 side leg lifts? (see page 52) | 5 |
| ★ Can you lift 1.5 kg (3 lbs) in a wrist curl? (see page 64) | 5 |

Note your score and chart your improvements

DATE          TOTAL SCORE =

## WHAT WAS YOUR SCORE?

★ You are safe to do all the home exercises if you scored 25 or over in 'Did you', and 40 or over in 'Can you'.

★ If your scores were below this, choose the gentler versions of the exercises and progress slowly.

★ If your score was below 7 in 'Did you', and below 15 in 'Can you', then start with the good practice section, balance exercises, walking, stair climbing and aquaerobics.

# TAILOR YOUR OWN PROGRAMME

There are more exercises in this book than you could complete in one session, so choose the ones which will be most useful to you, and vary them from time to time.

Each exercise takes about 5 minutes for 3 sets of 8 lifts, and the double exercises (left + right side) take about 6 minutes, so you can do 6 single or 4 double exercises in a 40 minute session, in addition to preparation, warm-up, stretching and relaxing. Later on, you can fit in more exercises by combining them (see 'For experienced exercisers'). Here are some ideas to help you plan. Don't forget your daily half dozen (see pages 20–23).

## Planning your session
Always include these elements:
★ Prepare your space and warm-up
★ Balance exercises
★ Home exercises
★ Stretch and relax

## For beginners or older women
Begin with these eight home exercises, which do not need any equipment. Add a few new ones week by week.

★ **Monday**    Back Lift
                     Side Leg Lift
                     Arm Press
                     Straight Leg Lift

★ **Wednesday**    Aquaerobics or
                     T'ai Chi

★ **Friday**    Leg Lift
                     Abdominal Lift
                     All-fours
                     Thigh Lift

**OR**

On three separated days of the week, work through the stages of the walk–jog programme (see page 86) and do the Wrist Press, Twist & Pull exercises (see page 76). Take a stout walking stick and a friend and do it all in the park.

## For experienced exercisers
You can save time during your workout by combining exercises which use different muscle groups instead of resting between sets. For example, combine the Flying Back Lift and Chest Press:

★ **Flying Back Lift**
Do 8 lifts, roll over, then pick up dumb-bells

★ **Chest Press**
Do 8 lifts, put down dumb-bells, and roll over to do Flying Back Lifts again.

For double exercises, do 16 lifts (left + right side) of the first exercise then change over.
Other good pairings are:
★ Shoulder Press + Arm Curl
★ Back Lift + All-fours
★ Abdominal Lift + Leg Lift
★ Straight Leg Lift + Standing Leg Curl
★ Thigh Lift + Leg Press

# Food for Strong Bones

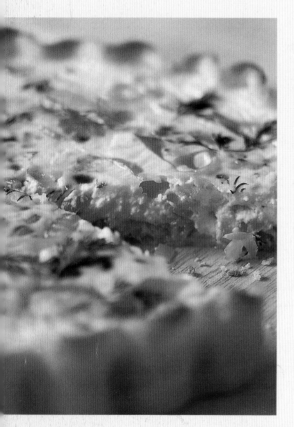

One of the most important ways in which we can develop and maintain strong bones is through a healthy diet; choosing a healthy, well balanced and varied diet that includes foods from each of the main food groups will help ensure a good intake of vitamins and minerals, especially calcium, which is essential for good bone health. Building strong bones when we are young and helping to reduce the effects of bone-density loss as we get older means that we can alleviate many of the symptoms of osteoporosis. This section features a wide variety of delicious recipes that have been devised to help you develop a diet that is great for strong, healthy bones and that will appeal to all the family. The recipes will also fit easily into your lifestyle, as the dishes are easy to prepare and all the ingredients are readily available in supermarkets.

## DIET AND OSTEOPOROSIS

Research has shown that a poor diet increases the risk of osteoporosis later in life. As we have seen, bones are made up of a thick outer shell with a strong, dense inner mesh that has a honeycomb-like structure. A good calcium intake is vital because this gives the bones their strength and rigidity. As bone becomes old it is removed by the body and replaced with new bone – it has been calculated that adults replace their entire skeletons every seven to 10 years. Calcium, therefore, gets deposited and withdrawn from the skeleton on a daily basis. As we get older, this renewal process slows down and bone-density loss increases. When this happens, the holes in the bone's inner mesh gradually become bigger and the bones become more fragile. However, by maximising bone mass early in life and by maintaining a healthy diet, we can reduce the effects of this process.

## CALCIUM FOR EVERYONE

It's never too early or too late to begin eating for strong bones. A good calcium intake during childhood, adolescence and early adulthood, while the bones are still growing, will help to protect your bones throughout life. As we move into later life, maintaining a calcium-rich diet is equally important, in order to reduce the effects of bone loss. Bone density begins to decrease around the age of 35, so it is essential to adopt and maintain a bone-friendly diet throughout life.

Pregnant women need a good calcium intake to provide for the calcium needs of their babies. People on low-fat diets also need to ensure they are not missing out on calcium-rich foods such as dairy products. It is important to remember that low-fat dairy products can still be a good source of calcium, because when fat is removed to make reduced or low-fat products, the calcium remains (in fact, pint for pint, skimmed milk contains slightly more calcium than whole milk). This is especially important for teenage girls, who are more likely to embark on low-fat diets at a time when good calcium intake is vital.

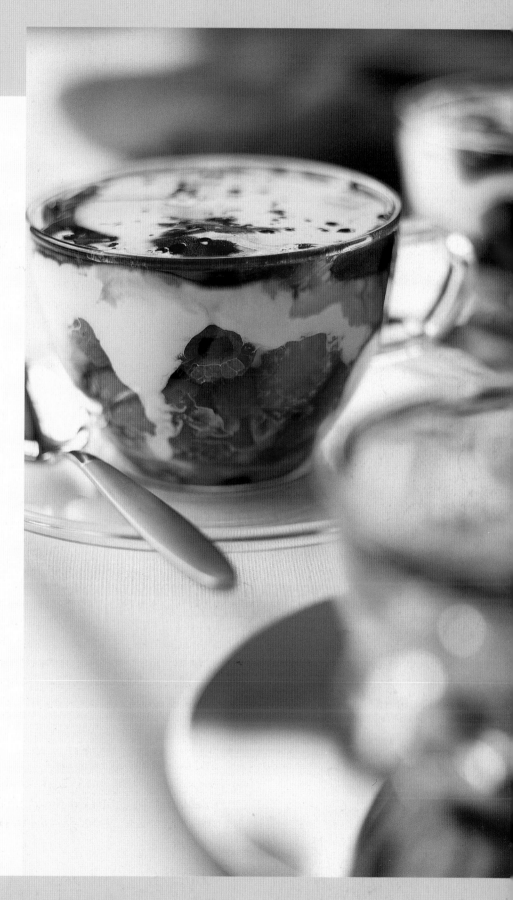

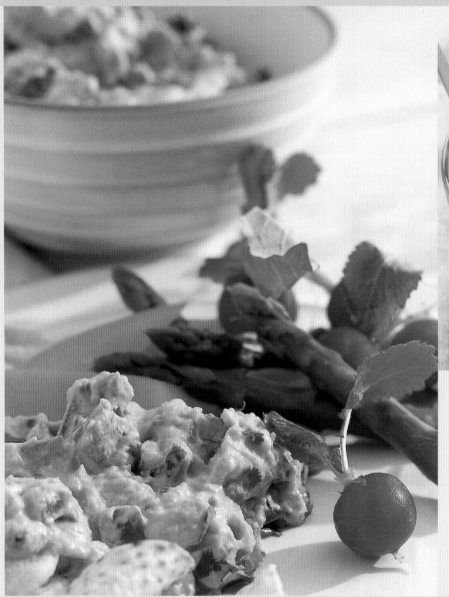

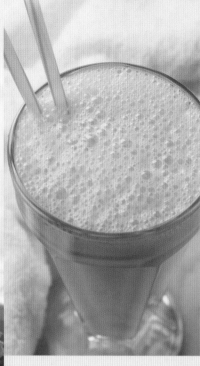

NUTRITIONAL ANALYSIS
See pages 218–221 for a
comprehensive nutritional
breakdown for each recipe.

RECOMMENDED DAILY INTAKES OF CALCIUM

| Age | Daily intake* | Number of servings** |
| --- | --- | --- |
| Children, 4–6 years | 450 mg | 2 |
| Children, 7–10 years | 550 mg | 2–3 |
| Boys, 11–18 years | 1000 mg | 3–4 |
| Girls, 11–18 years | 800 mg | 2–3 |
| Men and women, 19–50 years | 700 mg | 2–3 |
| Men and women, 50 years and over | 700 mg | 2–3 |
| Pregnant women | 700 mg | 2–3 |
| Breastfeeding women | 700 + 550 mg | 4–5 |

* Recommended figures from National Osteoporosis Society
** 1 serving = 1 glass of milk, 150 g yogurt or 40 g hard full-fat cheese.

## GOOD SOURCES OF CALCIUM AND VITAMIN D

**Calcium** The richest sources of calcium are milk, cheese, yogurt and other dairy products. Bread, dark green vegetables such as spinach and broccoli, beans and pulses, almonds and tinned salmon, pilchards and sardines (if you eat the bones) also contain calcium. Some brands of orange juice and most breakfast cereals have added calcium. Mineral water can often contain calcium – but for all foods check the list on the packet as the amounts vary.

**Vitamin D** Oily fish and seafood such as salmon, tuna, herring and shrimp are good sources, as are fish liver oils. Egg yolks and liver also contain benficial amounts, and margarines and breakfast cereals are often fortified with vitamin D.

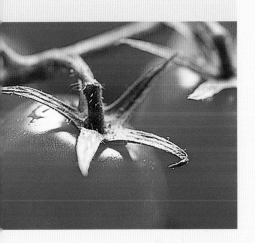

## BONE-FRIENDLY FOODS

As part of a diet for strong bones, and for your health in general, you need to eat a healthy, well balanced and varied diet that includes at least 5 servings of fruit and/or vegetables a day, plenty of wholegrain cereals and not too much sugar or fat. The following vitamins and minerals are particularly good for strong bones.

**Calcium** This is the most vital mineral for strong bones. Calcium is also essential for blood clotting, muscle contraction and nerve function and, if we don't take in enough, the body uses the calcium in the bones to supply the muscles, heart and nerves. In the average British diet, milk and other dairy products provide over 50 per cent of dietary calcium, and calcium is best absorbed into the body from milk and other dairy products. For other good food sources, see the box (*left*).

**Vitamin D** This is vital for the absorption of calcium and is produced when the skin is exposed to sunlight. About 15–20 minutes of sunlight a day on the face and arms during the summer months enables the body to store enough vitamin D to last the rest of the year. Most people obtain sufficient vitamin D in this way but some groups, such as the elderly or housebound, may have insufficient vitamin D. For good food sources of vitamin D see the box (*left*).

**Magnesium** Recent studies suggest that magnesium has an important role to play in helping to keep our bones healthy. Good sources of magnesium include Brazil nuts, sesame seeds, bananas, pine nuts, cashew nuts and dark green leafy vegetables, such as spinach and watercress.

**Vitamin K** Research shows that women who have a good intake of vitamin K have denser bones. Foods rich in vitamin K include curly kale, broccoli and spinach.

**Fruit and vegetables** There is growing evidence suggesting a positive link between eating plenty of fruit and vegetables and better bone density. Aim to eat at least five portions of fruit or vegetables a day.

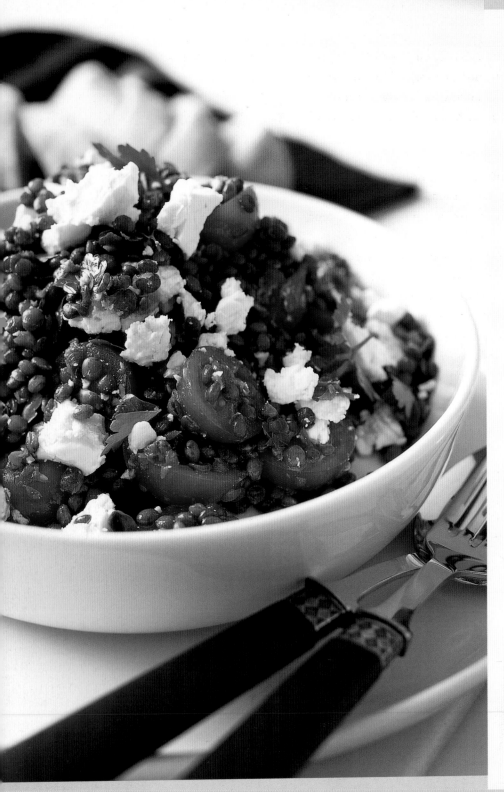

BE CAREFUL WITH . . .
**Protein** High intakes of protein increase the excretion of calcium in the urine. For most people, however, protein intakes are not high enough to give cause for concern, but it could be a problem if you take protein supplements or follow a high-protein, weight-reducing diet.

**Salt** High sodium (salt) intake can also increase the loss of calcium in the urine. Over three-quarters of the sodium in our diet comes from processed foods, so the simplest way to reduce sodium intake is to eat fewer processed foods. Food with less salt may initially taste bland, but by gradually reducing the amount of salt you eat, the tastebuds will adapt as the salt receptors on the tongue become more sensitive. Try using other flavourings such as herbs and spices, lemon or mustard.

**Caffeine** High intakes of caffeine can reduce absorption of calcium – each cup of coffee prevents the absorption of 6 mg of calcium, which is the amount you would get from 1 teaspoon of milk. The effect of caffeine is relatively small, but people with very high intakes should cut back.

**Alcohol** Excessive intakes of alcohol can damage the cells that make new bone. If you drink, stay within the recommended guidelines (no more than 2–3 units of alcohol a day for women or 3–4 units for men).

**Fizzy drinks** Phosphate, in the form of phosphoric acid, is used as a preservative in most canned fizzy drinks. When phosphorus levels exceed calcium levels in the blood, the body responds by stimulating bone breakdown to release calcium into the blood. Although there is no hard scientific evidence to show a detrimental effect on bone health, it is probably wise to cut back if you have an excessive intake, and to limit the amount of fizzy drinks your children consume. Instead, why not offer a glass of cold milk?

## NOTES TO THE COOK

To minimise the fat content of the dishes, all milk should be semi-skimmed, unless specified in the ingredients. Also, because a high sodium intake is not good for your bones, or your general health, the sodium content of the recipes has been kept as low as possible. If you do add salt, keep it to a minimum.

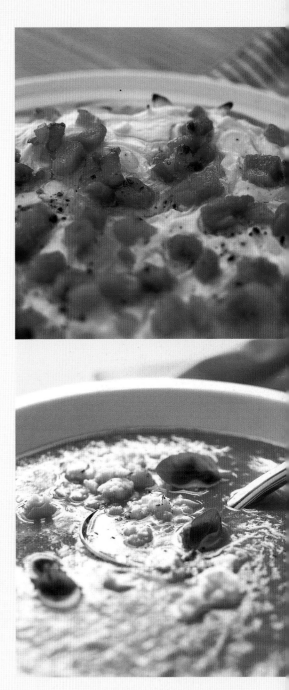

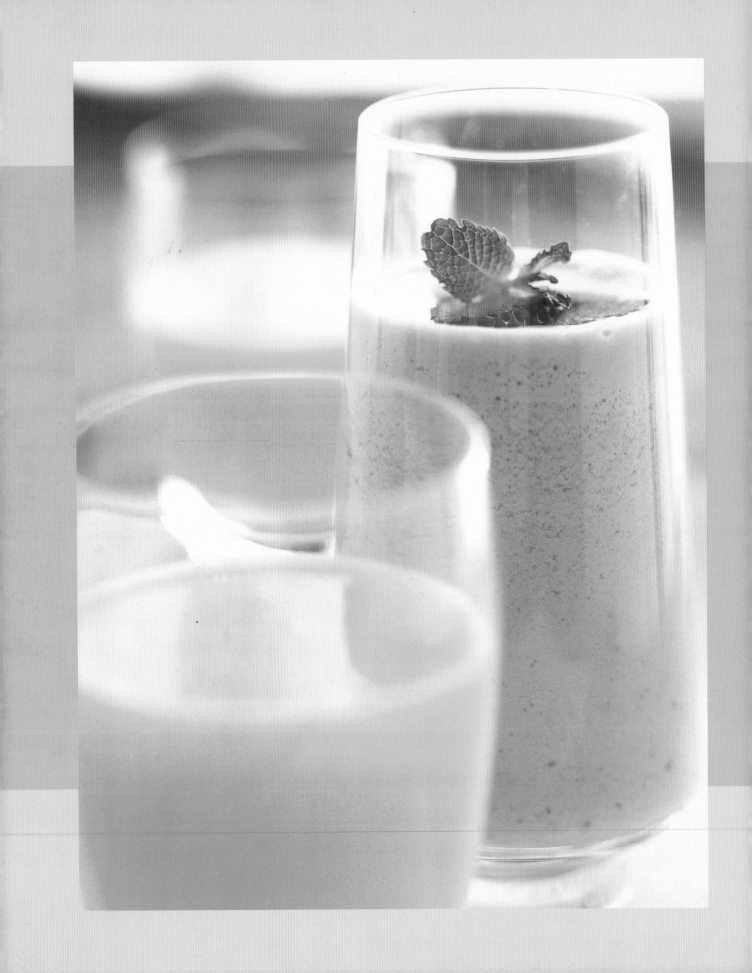

# 1
# Start the Day

Whether you prefer a sweet or savoury breakfast, this chapter offers a variety of calcium-rich recipes that will give you the best possible start to the day.

# SWEET FRUIT PORRIDGE

125 g raisins or chopped dried dates

150 ml water

150 ml milk

125 g rolled oats

Pinch of salt

Serves 4

*Extra sweetness is released from the dried fruit when it is liquidised, so you don't need to add any sugar or honey.*

1   In a blender or food processor, blend the raisins or chopped dates with the water and milk until smooth.

2   In a heavy based saucepan, combine the fruit mixture with the oats and add a pinch of salt. Bring to the boil, stirring steadily. Simmer the mixture, uncovered, stirring occasionally, for 4–5 minutes until the desired consistency is reached. Serve with extra milk, if liked.

# APPLE & BLUEBERRY MUESLI

5 tablespoons rolled oats

2 tablespoons sultanas

2 tablespoons flaked almonds

8 tablespoons apple juice

250 ml plain bio-yogurt

200 ml semi-skimmed milk

1 tablespoon clear honey

2 crisp eating apples, cored and grated

75 g fresh blueberries

Serves 2–3

*This muesli mix is packed full of delicious ingredients that are good for your bone health, and with none of the additives found in some commercially produced cereals. Soaking the oats in apple juice and milk gives this a fruity flavour, while keeping the calcium content high.*

1   Mix together the oats, sultanas, almonds and apple juice and allow to stand for a few minutes, until the juice is absorbed.

2   Stir the yogurt, milk, honey and grated apple into the oats and leave to stand for 15 minutes.

3   Stir in the blueberries and serve.

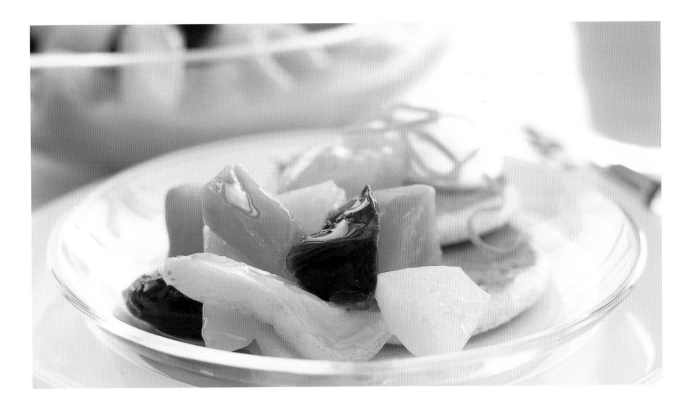

# SPICED FRUIT COMPOTE

*Dried fruits are useful source of calcium, particularly for people on dairy-free diets. They also make a tasty snack in between meals. This compote can also be served with natural yogurt as a dessert.*

1   Put the dried fruit, cinnamon stick and cardamon pods in a large bowl. Pour over the apple and mango juice and 450 ml of boiling water. Allow to cool, cover and leave overnight in the fridge.

2   Remove the cardamon pods and cinnamon stick. Mix the cornflour with enough cold water to make a smooth paste. Drain the liquid from the fruit and place in a small saucepan. Stir in the cornflour paste and bring to the boil. Cook for 1 minute, or until thickened, then pour over the compote. Set aside and leave to cool.

3   Place 2 Scotch pancakes on each of 4 plates with a large spoonful of the fruit compote and a large spoonful of Greek yogurt. Sprinkle with orange zest to serve.

250 g mixed ready-to-eat dried fruit, such as apricots, apples and prunes or papaya, mango and pineapple

1 stick cinnamon

3 whole green cardamom pods, lightly crushed

225 ml apple juice

225 ml mango juice

2 teaspoons cornflour

TO SERVE

8 ready-made Scotch pancakes

4 tablespoons Greek yogurt

Zest of 1 orange

Serves 4

# DRIED FRUIT SPREAD

175 g ready-to-eat dried apricots, roughly chopped

175 g dried figs, roughly chopped

75 g ready-to-eat dried apple, roughly chopped

Zest of 1 orange

200 ml unsweetened orange juice

Makes 450 g (about 25 portions)

*This is a healthier alternative to jam or marmalade and is delicious spread on warm, buttered toast. You could also try stirring a tablespoon of the spread into low-fat plain yogurt. It will keep for 3 weeks if stored in jars in the fridge.*

1   Place the apricots, figs, apple, orange zest and juice into a pan and bring to the boil. Reduce the heat and simmer for 20–30 minutes, or until the mixture is thick and the orange juice has evaporated. You can add a little more orange juice if necessary, but the final purée should be quite thick.

2   Transfer the mixture to a blender and purée until smooth. Spoon the purée into jars and store in the fridge.

# BAGELS WITH RASPBERRIES & RICOTTA

100 g fresh raspberries

75 g ricotta cheese

1 tablespoon icing sugar

2 cinnamon or fruit bagels, halved

Serves 2

*Ricotta cheese contains a lot less fat than most other creamy cheeses, but still provides useful amounts of calcium.*

1   Place the raspberries, ricotta and icing sugar in a bowl and mash until combined. Place in the fridge until needed.

2   Lightly toast the bagels and spread over the raspberry and ricotta mixture.

# BANANA & ALMOND SMOOTHIE

2 ripe bananas

450 ml semi-skimmed milk

40 g ground almonds

1–2 teaspoons honey, to sweeten (optional)

Serves 2

*The combination of milk and fruit in smoothies is great for strong bones. Almonds are an excellent source of vitamin E, along with the minerals calcium, magnesium, phosphorus and copper. They also give this smoothie a rich, creamy taste.*

1   Peel and slice the bananas, place in a freezer-proof container and freeze for at least 2 hours, or overnight.

2   Place the bananas, milk, almonds and honey in a blender or food processor and blend until thick and frothy. Pour into glasses and serve immediately.

# APRICOT & ORANGE SMOOTHIE

*Both dried apricots and orange juice are useful sources of calcium,
making this a good alternative to milk-based smoothies
for people on dairy-free diets.*

1  Place the apricots in a small saucepan and pour over 300 ml water.
Bring to the boil and simmer over a low heat for 10 minutes, or until the
apricots are soft.

2  Place the apricots and any remaining water in a liquidiser. Pour in the
orange juice and purée until smooth.

3  To serve, pour into glasses and add a couple of ice cubes to serve.

125 g ready-to-eat dried apricots,
chopped into small pieces

400 ml orange juice

Serves 2

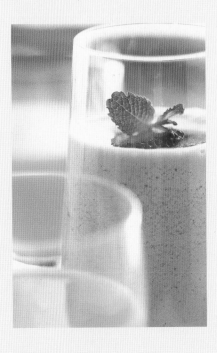

# STRAWBERRY SMOOTHIE

*Strawberries are rich in vitamin C, which is needed for healthy
bones. The fortified soya milk is a good non-dairy alternative
to cow's milk and also adds vital calcium.*

1  Switch the freezer to 'fast freeze'. Roughly chop the strawberries and place
in a plastic freezerproof container. Freeze for at least 2 hours, or preferably
overnight. If your freezer does not have a 'fast freeze' function, you will
need to freeze the strawberries overnight.

2  Remove the strawberry pieces from the freezer and turn the freezer setting
back to 'normal', if necessary. Reserve about 200 g of the strawberry pieces
to decorate, then purée the remainder in a food processor or blender with
the soya milk until smooth.

3  Pour the smoothie into 4 large glasses and decorate with the remaining
strawberries. Garnish with mint sprigs to serve.

750 g fresh ripe strawberries

600 ml sweetened calcium-fortified
soya milk

Fresh mint sprigs, to garnish

Serves 4

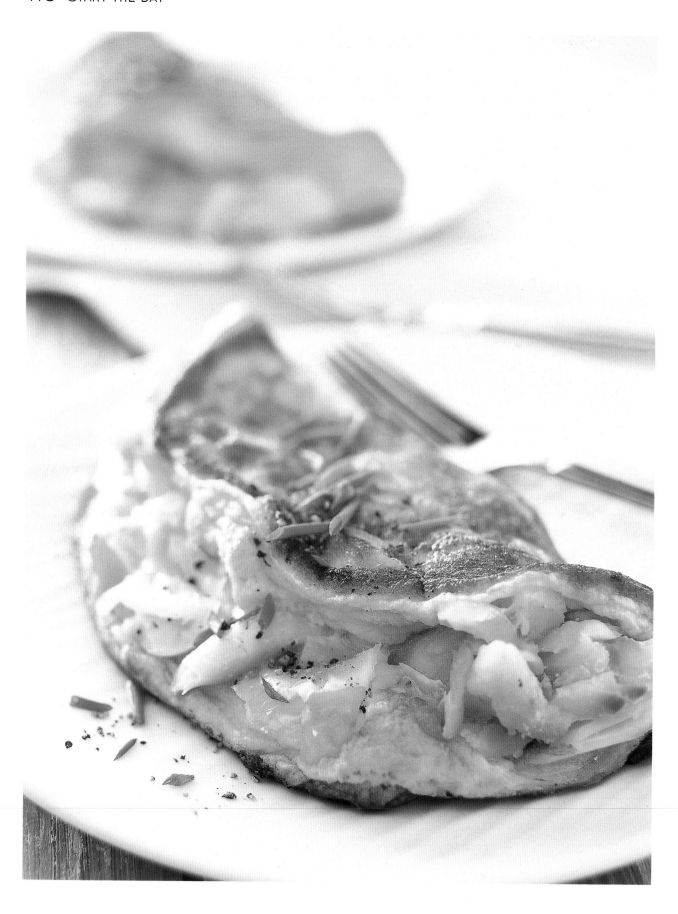

# CHEESY SCRAMBLED EGGS

*This breakfast provides a perfect combination of ingredients for strong bones – cheese is rich in calcium while the eggs provide vitamin D, which is essential for optimum calcium absorption.*

1  Mix the eggs and milk together and season to taste. Heat the butter in a non-stick saucepan. Add the eggs and cook over a low heat, stirring continuously.

2  Once the eggs are scrambled, remove from the heat and stir in the cheese and spring onions. Serve immediately on wholemeal toast.

4 eggs, beaten

2 tablespoons semi-skimmed milk

Salt and pepper, to taste

1 teaspoon butter

50 g Cheddar cheese, grated

4 spring onions, finely chopped

Wholemeal toast, to serve

Serves 2

# SMOKED HADDOCK OMELETTE

*This omelette is a substantial, nutritious breakfast that is still quick and easy to make.*

1  Place the fish in a shallow pan and cover with water. Bring to the boil, reduce the heat and simmer gently for 5 minutes, or until the fish is cooked. Drain, then flake the fish, discarding the skin and bones.

2  Preheat the grill. Beat the egg yolks in a bowl with the milk and seasoning. Stir in the flaked fish. Whisk the egg whites until stiff then, using a metal spoon, fold into the yolk mixture.

3  Heat the butter in an omelette pan. Pour in the egg mixture and cook for 2–3 minutes or until the bottom of the omelette is set. Slide the omelette onto a flameproof serving dish.

4  Sprinkle over the cheese and place under the grill for 2–3 minutes, or until the top has set and the cheese melted. Garnish with chives to serve.

125 g smoked haddock

4 eggs, separated

2 tablespoons full-fat milk

Salt and pepper, to taste

15 g butter

40 g Gruyère cheese, grated

Fresh chives, chopped, to garnish

Serves 2

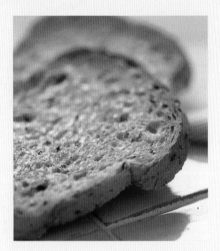

# SOFT EGGS WITH SOURED CREAM & SMOKED SALMON

*This is a special treat for breakfast or brunch, or a tasty and nutritious snack at any time. Both eggs and smoked salmon provide useful amounts of vitamin D, which helps the absorption of calcium. However, if you are serving this dish to anyone elderly, a pregnant woman, young children or people who have immune deficiency disease, boil the eggs for slightly longer, to make sure that they are well-cooked. This will eliminate any risk of salmonella.*

4 eggs

100 g smoked salmon

200 ml soured cream

1 teaspoon black peppercorns

2 punnets mustard and cress, to garnish

4 slices Granary toast, buttered, to serve

Serves 4

1 Lower the eggs into a pan of simmering water, making sure that the water covers them completely. Cook for 3½–5 minutes until soft-boiled. Drain and rinse under cool running water, until the eggs are cool enough to handle, then shell.

2 Meanwhile, chop roughly the smoked salmon and stir into the soured cream. Crack the black peppercorns, using a pestle and mortar. If you don't have a pestle and mortar, grind the peppercorns as coarsely as you can.

3 Halve the eggs and arrange on individual serving plates. Spoon over the smoked salmon and soured cream mixture. Scatter with the cracked black peppercorns and garnish with mustard and cress. Serve with buttered Granary toast.

# SMOKED HADDOCK & SWEETCORN FRITTERS

*Serve these light and tasty fritters with grilled tomatoes for a balanced and nutritious start to the day.*

1 Place the haddock in a shallow pan and pour over the milk. Bring to the boil, then cover and simmer for 6–7 minutes, or until the fish is cooked. Remove the fish from the milk, discard the skin and bones and flake the fish. Strain the milk and reserve.

2 Place the flour in a large bowl and make a well in the centre. Whisk in the egg yolk and enough of the reserved milk to make a thick batter (you should need about 125 ml). Stir in the sweetcorn and haddock and season to taste. In a clean bowl, whisk the egg white until it forms soft peaks, then carefully fold into the batter.

3 Cook the mixture in batches by dropping spoonfuls onto a lightly greased griddle or heavy based frying pan. Cook for 2–3 minutes, then turn carefully and cook for a further 2–3 minutes, until golden brown. Serve with the grilled tomatoes.

200 g smoked haddock

175 ml semi-skimmed milk

100 g plain flour

1 egg, separated

125 g canned sweetcorn, drained

Salt and pepper, to taste

Vegetable oil, for frying

6 grilled tomatoes, halved, to serve

Serves 4 (makes 8 fritters)

# STUFFED PORTOBELLO MUSHROOMS

*Mushrooms are often part of breakfast dishes, and this recipe uses them in a creative and interesting way. This is a tasty and satisfying breakfast or brunch that takes just a few minutes to prepare. Serve with buttered Granary toast.*

1 Preheat the oven to 220°C, gas mark 7. Wipe the mushrooms with a damp cloth, then remove and finely chop the stalks. Lightly brush the cap of each mushroom with a little olive oil and place on a baking sheet.

2 Heat the remaining oil in a large non-stick frying pan and add the chopped mushroom stalks, onions and celery. Cook over a medium heat, stirring occasionally, for 3–4 minutes, or until the vegetables are beginning to soften.

3 Stir in the breadcrumbs, ham, parsley and lemon zest, then season with salt and pepper.

4 Spoon the breadcrumb mixture into the mushrooms then sprinkle with the Parmesan cheese. Bake in the oven for 15–20 minutes, or until the mushrooms are tender and golden. Garnish with sprigs of flat-leaf parsley.

8 Portobello (large flat) mushrooms

2 tablespoons olive oil

1 medium red onion, finely chopped

6 sticks celery, finely chopped

150 g fine white breadcrumbs

225 g wafer-thin smoked ham, roughly chopped

6 tablespoons fresh flat-leaf parsley, chopped

Zest of 1 large lemon

Salt and pepper, to taste

3 tablespoons Parmesan cheese, freshly grated

Sprigs of flat-leaf parsley, to garnish

Serves 4

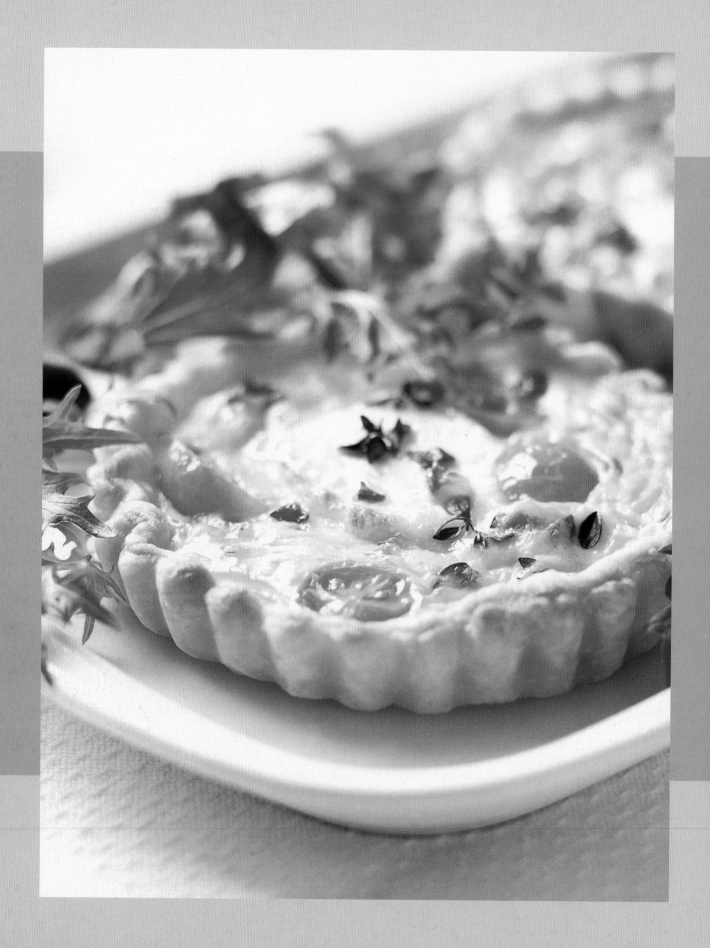

# 2

# Soups & Starters

THE DISHES IN THIS CHAPTER MAKE
THE MOST OF BOTH DAIRY AND NON-
DAIRY SOURCES OF CALCIUM AND
OTHER VITAMINS AND MINERALS. MANY
OF THE RECIPES CAN BE PREPARED IN
ADVANCE AND SERVED WHEN
REQUIRED.

# BROCCOLI & STILTON SOUP

*Broccoli is an excellent source of calcium and vitamin C, so is ideal as part of a bone-friendly diet. Serve this soup with crusty bread.*

1 tablespoon vegetable oil

1 medium onion, finely chopped

1 clove garlic, peeled and finely chopped

1 large floury potato, such as Maris Piper, peeled and finely diced

600 ml vegetable stock

450 g broccoli, trimmed and roughly chopped

300 ml semi-skimmed milk

Salt and pepper, to taste

125 g Stilton, crumbled

Serves 4–6

1   Heat the oil in large pan, then add the onion and garlic and cook for 3–4 minutes. Add the potato and continue to cook, stirring occasionally, for 2–3 minutes.

2   Add the stock and bring to the boil, then reduce the heat, cover and cook for 10 minutes. Add the broccoli and simmer for 5–10 minutes, or until the broccoli is just tender.

3   Place the mixture in a blender and purée until smooth, then return to the pan. Stir in the milk, season to taste and gently reheat. When the soup is hot, stir in the Stilton and, once the cheese has melted into the soup, serve.

# MOROCCAN SPICED CHICKPEA SOUP

*This wholesome soup is the perfect way to keep warm on a cold day. Chickpeas, along with other beans and pulses, are a useful source of calcium, particularly for people who don't eat dairy products.*

2 tablespoons olive oil

1 large onion, chopped

1 clove garlic, peeled and finely chopped

2 medium carrots, thickly sliced

2 sticks celery, thickly sliced

2 courgettes, thickly sliced

2 teaspoons ground cumin

1 teaspoon turmeric

1 tablespoon tomato purée

400 g can chopped tomatoes

400 g can chickpeas, drained

600 ml vegetable stock

3 tablespoons fresh coriander, chopped, to garnish

Serves 4

1   Heat the oil in a large non-stick pan and cook the onion and garlic for 5 minutes until soft.

2   Add the carrots, celery and courgettes and cook for a further 4–5 minutes, stirring occasionally.

3   Add the cumin and turmeric and stir to coat the vegetables. Add the tomato purée, canned tomatoes, chickpeas and stock. Bring to the boil then cover and simmer for 20–30 minutes, until the vegetables are soft. Garnish with fresh coriander and serve.

# ROASTED PEPPER SOUP WITH FETA & BASIL

*The roasted peppers give a subtle sweet flavour to this soup which is enhanced by the feta and basil. To save time, you could substitute cans or jars of roasted peppers or sweet pimentos.*

1   Preheat the oven to 200°C, gas mark 6. Put the pepper halves cut-side down on a large baking sheet and roast for 25–30 minutes or until the skins are blackened. Leave to cool slightly then put the peppers into a polythene bag for 10 minutes, until the skins loosen. Remove the skins, chop the flesh roughly and set aside.

2   Heat the oil in large saucepan and cook the onion and garlic for 5 minutes, until soft. Add the chopped peppers, tomatoes, vegetable stock and seasoning. Bring to the boil, cover and simmer for 20 minutes. Remove from the heat and purée the soup in a blender or processor (you will probably need to do this in batches). Return to the pan, add the shredded basil and reheat.

3   To serve, spoon into soup bowls and scatter over the feta. Garnish with basil leaves and a grinding of black pepper.

4 large red peppers, halved, cored and deseeded or 450 g jar roasted red peppers, drained and rinsed

2 tablespoons olive oil

1 large red onion, roughly chopped

2 cloves garlic, peeled and roughly chopped

400 g can chopped tomatoes

900 ml vegetable stock

Salt and pepper, to taste

2 tablespoons fresh basil, shredded

100 g feta cheese, crumbled

Fresh basil leaves, to garnish

Serves 6

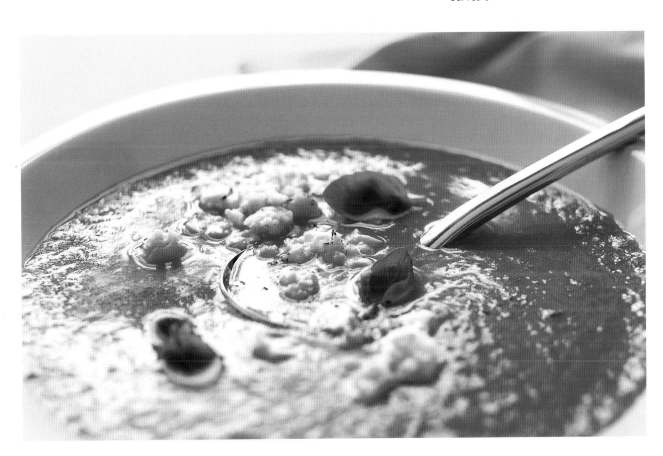

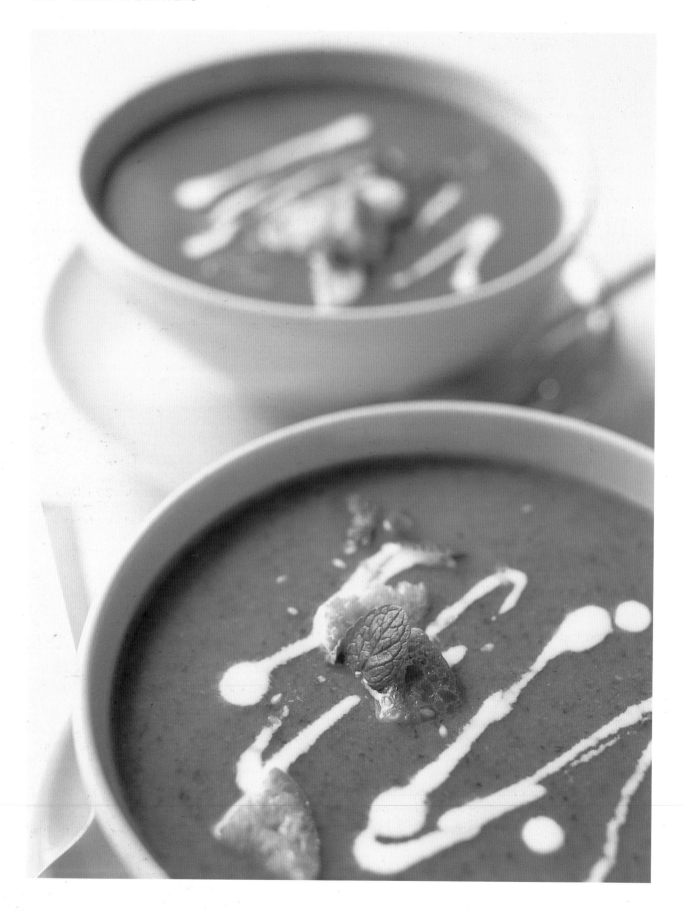

# FRENCH ONION SOUP

*Here, this traditional soup is served ladled over toasted bread with a sprinkling of Gruyère cheese. For a change, the Gruyère can be replaced with goat's cheese, Emmenthal, mozzarella or any blue cheese.*

1 Melt the butter in a large saucepan, add the onions and cook gently for 15–20 minutes until they are golden brown.

2 Sift the flour into the pan and cook, stirring continuously, for 1 minute. Stir in the stock, seasoning and add the bay leaf. Bring to the boil, cover and simmer for 30 minutes.

3 Cut the French loaf diagonally into 1 cm slices. Heat the grill to medium and toast the bread lightly on both sides. Place two slices in each of 4 ovenproof soup bowls and ladle over the hot soup, discarding the bay leaf.

4 Turn the grill to high. Sprinkle the Gruyère cheese over the soup and place under the grill until the cheese is melted and bubbling. Serve immediately.

50 g butter

3 large onions, thinly sliced

1 tablespoon plain flour

900 ml vegetable stock

Salt and pepper, to taste

1 bay leaf

½ medium French loaf

75 g Gruyère cheese, grated

Serves 4

# GARDEN PEA & WATERCRESS SOUP WITH SESAME CROUTONS

*The bright colour of this creamy, fresh-tasting soup makes it an eye-catching starter, while the sesame croutons add texture.*

1 To make the croutons, brush the ciabatta pieces with 2 tablespoons of the oil and sprinkle with the sesame seeds. Heat the remaining oil in a non-stick pan and cook the croutons over a high heat for 3–4 minutes until crisp and golden. Remove and drain on kitchen paper, then set aside to cool.

2 To make the soup, melt the butter in a large saucepan. Add the onion and cook for 5 minutes until soft, then add the peas, watercress, stock and seasoning. Bring slowly to the boil, lower the heat, cover and simmer for 5 minutes.

3 Allow the soup to cool slightly, then process in a blender or food processor until smooth (you will probably need to do this in batches). Pour into a clean saucepan, season to taste and reheat.

4 Drizzle with crème fraîche and garnish with chopped mint and the sesame croutons. Serve with chunks of wholemeal or granary bread.

**FOR THE SESAME CROUTONS**

3 slices ciabatta bread, cut into small pieces

3 tablespoons olive oil

1 tablespoon sesame seeds

**FOR THE SOUP**

40 g butter

1 large onion, finely chopped

450 g fresh or frozen peas

75 g fresh watercress, roughly chopped

1 litre hot vegetable stock

Salt and pepper, to taste

4–6 tablespoons crème fraîche, to garnish

Fresh mint leaves, to garnish

Serves 4–6

# Smoked Haddock & Sweetcorn Chowder

25 g butter

1 medium onion, peeled and finely chopped

2 medium floury potatoes, such as Maris Piper, peeled and cut into small cubes

400 ml fish stock

300 g canned sweetcorn, drained

400 ml semi-skimmed milk

450 g skinless smoked haddock fillets, cut into bite-sized pieces

Salt and pepper, to taste

Fresh parsley, chopped, to garnish

Serves 4

*Using semi-skimmed milk gives this soup a creamy rich taste, while reducing the fat content of the dish. It is also a good source of calcium. The soup is delicious served with crusty bread.*

1  Melt the butter in a large saucepan, add the onion and cook over a gentle heat for 5 minutes until soft. Add the potato and continue cooking for a further 2 minutes.

2  Add the fish stock and bring to the boil. Reduce the heat, cover and simmer for about 10–15 minutes, or until the potatoes are tender. Roughly mash the potatoes.

3  Add the sweetcorn and milk and return to the boil. Reduce the heat and simmer for 5 minutes. Stir in the fish and continue to cook for a further 5 minutes. Season to taste and garnish with chopped parsley.

# Baked Ricotta with Roasted Vine Tomatoes

Butter, for greasing

300 g ricotta cheese

125 g Parmesan cheese, freshly grated

2 eggs, separated

Salt and pepper, to taste

4 plum tomatoes, halved

1 tablespoon olive oil

1 tablespoon balsamic vinegar

Serves 4

*This dish is ideal as a starter or a light lunch with a green salad. Mixing Parmesan cheese with the ricotta cheese boosts the flavour as well as the calcium content.*

1  Preheat the oven to 180°C, gas mark 4. Grease a shallow ovenproof dish.

2  Place the ricotta and Parmesan cheeses in a bowl and beat in the egg yolks until the mixture is smooth. Season to taste.

3  In a clean bowl, beat the egg whites until stiff. Using a metal spoon, fold the egg whites into the cheese mixture.

4  Spoon the mixture into the prepared dish and bake for 30–40 minutes, or until slightly risen, golden and firm to the touch. Allow to cool.

5  Place the tomatoes cut-side up on a baking tray. Mix the olive oil and balsamic vinegar together and drizzle over the tomatoes. Season and bake for 20 minutes, or until the tomatoes are softened and slightly charred.

6  Slice the baked cheese into quarters and serve with the tomatoes.

# MUSHROOMS & GOAT'S CHEESE IN AUBERGINE PARCELS

*These tasty parcels are ideal as a starter, and a rocket salad with balsamic dressing makes a good accompaniment. Mushrooms are rich in copper, which is a vital mineral for strong bones.*

1 Cut the aubergine lengthways into thin slices. Sprinkle with salt and set aside for 30 minutes. Rinse well and pat dry with kitchen roll. Brush the aubergine with 1 tablespoon oil and place under a hot grill for 2–3 minutes on each side, until golden brown. Transfer to a plate lined with kitchen paper and set to one side.

2 Heat the remaining oil in large non-stick frying pan, add the garlic, spring onions and mushrooms and cook for 10–15 minutes, until all the liquid has evaporated. Set to one side to cool.

3 Combine the mushroom mixture and the goat's cheese and season to taste. Line the base and sides of two 150 ml ramekin dishes with the grilled aubergine slices, allowing about one third of the slices to hang over the edge. Spoon the mushroom and cheese mixture into the ramekins and fold over the aubergine slices to encase the mixture.

4 Chill for 15 minutes, then turn the parcels out onto a lightly oiled baking sheet. Cook at 190°C, gas mark 5 for 10–15 minutes and serve immediately.

|  |
| --- |
| 1 long, thin aubergine |
| Salt, for sprinkling aubergine |
| 2 tablespoons olive oil |
| 1 clove garlic, peeled and finely chopped |
| 4 spring onions, finely chopped |
| 150 g button mushrooms, finely chopped |
| 125 g soft goat's cheese, rind removed |
| Salt and pepper, to taste |
| Serves 2 |

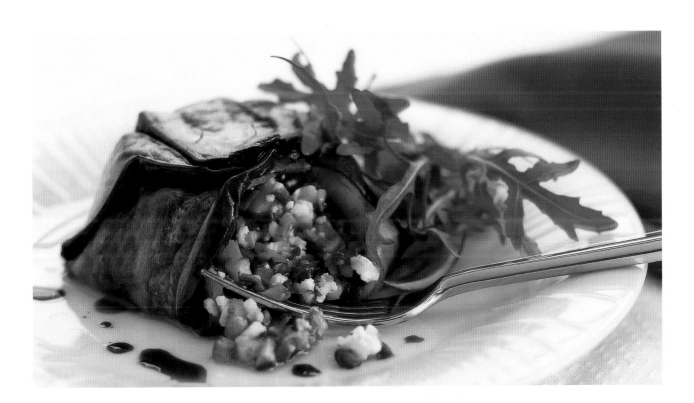

# CHERRY TOMATO & GOAT'S CHEESE TARTLETS

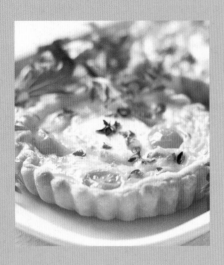

*These crisp individual pastry cases have a rich cheese and tomato filling and make a great starter. They also make a delicious lunchtime snack, accompanied by a leafy green salad.*

1 Preheat the oven to 200°C, gas mark 6. On a lightly floured surface, roll out the puff pastry and use to line four 10 cm tartlet tins. Line the pastry cases with baking parchment and fill with baking beans. Chill for 10 minutes.

2 Bake the pastry cases for 10 minutes. Remove the paper and beans and bake for a further 10 minutes, until the pastry is lightly golden.

3 Meanwhile, heat the oil in a non-stick frying pan. Add the red onion and thyme. Cook gently for 3–4 minutes until soft. Remove from the heat and set aside.

4 Beat the eggs and cream together. Add the Gruyère cheese and cooled onion mixture. Season and mix well. Cut the goat's cheese into 4 round slices. Divide the egg mixture between the tartlets and put 4 cherry tomato halves and 1 goat's cheese slice in each tartlet.

5 Bake the tartlets for 15 minutes until the filling is set. Cool slightly before removing them from the tins. Scatter a few thyme leaves over the warm tartlets just before serving.

Flour, for dusting

225 g ready-made puff pastry

1 tablespoon olive oil

1 medium red onion, finely chopped

1 teaspoon fresh thyme, chopped

2 eggs

150 ml single cream

25 g Gruyère cheese, finely grated

Salt and pepper, to taste

100 g firm, round goat's cheese

8 cherry tomatoes, halved

Few fresh thyme leaves, to garnish

Serves 4

# TOMATO & MOZZARELLA SALAD

*A classic combination which makes a tasty starter or a welcome accompaniment to most Italian dishes. If you're watching your fat intake, choose reduced-fat mozzarella cheese; although it contains less fat, it is still a good source of calcium. Serve with crusty bread.*

1 Whisk together the oil and vinegar to make the dressing. Season to taste.

2 Arrange the tomatoes and mozzarella cheese on a large plate. Drizzle over the dressing and scatter the basil over the top.

6 tablespoons olive oil

2 tablespoons white wine vinegar

Salt and pepper, to taste

3 large beefsteak tomatoes, thickly sliced

2 x 150 g round mozzarella cheeses, thickly sliced

24 leaves fresh basil, roughly torn

Serves 4–6

# WATERCRESS, PEAR & ROQUEFORT SALAD

*The contrasting flavours in this salad make it an interesting snack, starter or accompaniment. Roquefort, watercress and almonds are all rich in bone-strengthening calcium. Serve with crusty bread.*

1   To make the dressing, whisk together the oil, vinegar, mustard and salt.

2   Place the watercress in a large serving bowl. Peel, core and slice the pears and mix into the watercress, along with the cheese and almonds. Drizzle over the dressing and toss.

## FOR THE DRESSING

5 tablespoons olive oil

1 tablespoon white wine vinegar

½ teaspoon English mustard powder

Pinch of salt

## FOR THE SALAD

150 g watercress, washed

2 ripe pears

200 g Roquefort cheese, crumbled

50 g flaked almonds, lightly toasted

Serves 4

# AVOCADO & SMOKED SALMON ROLLS

*Reduced-fat soft cheese contains considerably less fat than full-fat cheese, but still contains good amounts of calcium. Oil-rich fish, such as salmon, provide vitamin D which is essential for the absorption of calcium. These rolls are delicious served with wholemeal toast.*

1   Remove the flesh of the avocado and mash. Add the cheese, lemon juice and seasoning and mix well. Chill the mixture in the fridge for 15 minutes.

2   Place the strips of salmon on a sheet of greaseproof paper and spread with the avocado mixture. Roll the salmon, from the shortest side, to enclose the avocado. Wrap the salmon rolls in greaseproof paper and place in the fridge until needed – they can prepared up to 4 hours in advance. To serve, garnish with lemon wedges.

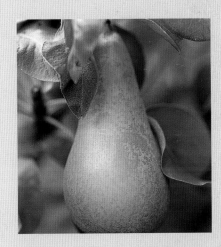

1 medium-ripe avocado

125 g reduced-fat soft cheese

Juice of half a lemon

Salt and pepper, to taste

125 g smoked salmon, cut into 4 strips, each about 12 × 9 cm

Lemon wedges, to garnish

Serves 2

# Roasted Red Pepper Dip

2 large red peppers, halved

125 g quark or reduced-fat soft cheese

2 teaspoons sweet chilli sauce

Salt and pepper, to taste

Serves 2–3

*This delicious red pepper dip is ideal for serving with crudités, but for a tasty, nutritious lunchtime snack, it can be spread on wholemeal bread and topped with a few salad leaves or alfalfa sprouts.*

1  Preheat the oven to 200°C, gas mark 6. Put the pepper halves cut-side down on a large baking sheet and roast for 25–30 minutes, or until the skins are blackened. Leave to cool slightly then put into a polythene bag for 10 minutes, until the skins loosen. Peel away the skin, chop the flesh roughly and set aside.

2  Place the peppers, quark or soft cheese, chilli sauce and seasoning into a food processor or blender and process for 1–2 minutes, until smooth.

3  Cover and place in the fridge for at least 2 hours before serving to allow the flavours to develop.

# Tzatziki

½ large cucumber

200 ml Greek yogurt

1 clove garlic, peeled and finely chopped

Salt and pepper, to taste

Serves 2–3

*Tzatziki makes a delicious lower-fat alternative to creamy dips and sauces. Serve with vegetable crudités and strips of warm pitta bread.*

1  Slice the cucumber in half lengthways. Deseed and dice the flesh.

2  Mix the yogurt, cucumber, garlic and seasoning together. Cover and set aside until needed.

# Creamy Guacamole

4 ripe avocados

3 plum tomatoes, skinned, deseeded and diced

Juice of 1 lime

1 clove garlic, peeled and finely chopped

6 tablespoons Greek yogurt

1 large red chilli, deseeded and chopped (optional)

2 tablespoons fresh coriander, chopped

Salt and pepper, to taste

Serves 6

*It is essential to use ripe avocados when making guacamole – they should 'give' slightly when pressed at the pointed end. A hard, under-ripe fruit will ripen in 1–2 days at room temperature, if stored in a bowl with ripe fruit. Serve with ready-made tortilla chips and crisp vegetable sticks.*

1  Cut the avocados in half and remove the stones. Using a spoon, scoop the flesh into a bowl and mash thoroughly.

2  Add the tomatoes, lime juice, garlic, yogurt, red chilli (if using), coriander and seasoning. Cover the bowl with clingfilm to prevent discolouring, making sure there are no gaps. Chill for 1–2 hours.

3  Uncover and mix lightly once more before serving.

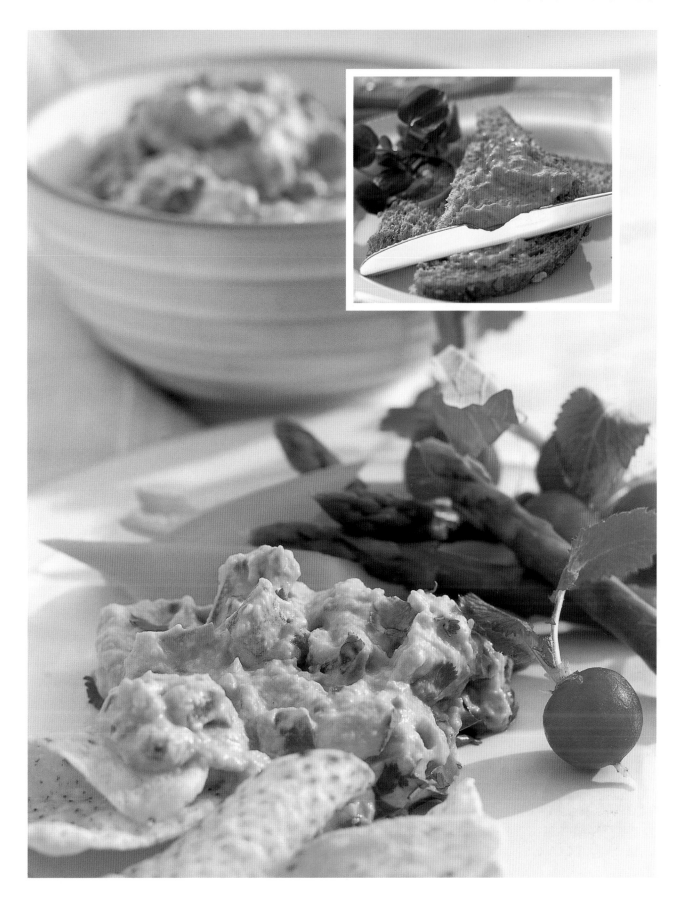

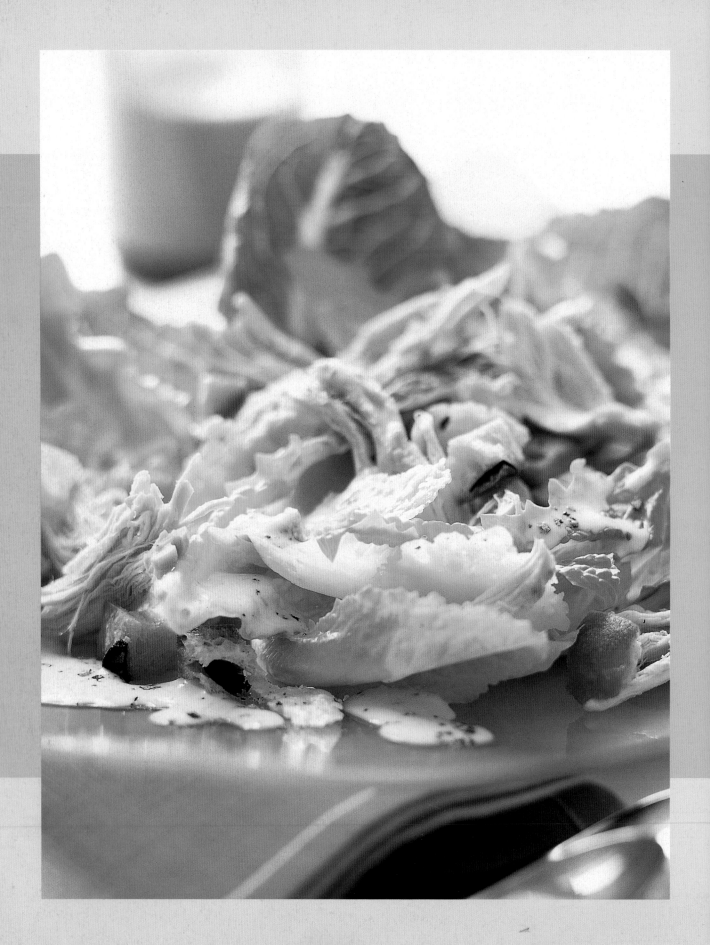

# 3

# Light Snacks & Lunches

It's easy to resort to ready-made, processed foods when we want a snack, but these often contain many unwanted additives and very few vitamins and minerals. This chapter offers quick and easy-to-prepare snacks and lunches that are both appealing and healthy.

# HUMOUS

400 g can chickpeas, drained and rinsed

2 tablespoons lemon juice

1 teaspoon ground cumin

50 ml extra virgin olive oil, plus extra for drizzling

2 cloves garlic, peeled

4 tablespoons tahini

Cayenne pepper, for dusting

Vegetable crudités or toasted pitta bread, to serve

Serves 4

*Home-made humous is quick and easy to prepare and knocks spots off the shop-bought variety. Cans of chickpeas are a nutritious and versatile store cupboard ingredient – apart from using them to make humous, you can add them to salads, soups, stews and casseroles.*

1 Put the chickpeas in a food processor or blender and process until semi-smooth. Add the lemon juice, cumin, oil, garlic and tahini and continue to blend until smooth. If the mixture is too thick, add a little more oil.

2 Place the mixture in a bowl, spoon over a little extra virgin oil and dust with cayenne or paprika. Serve immediately with vegetable crudités or toasted pitta, or cover and chill until needed.

# RED PEPPER HUMOUS

2 large red peppers

400 g can chickpeas, drained and rinsed

2 tablespoons lemon juice

1 teaspoon sweet chilli sauce

50 ml extra virgin olive oil

2 cloves garlic, peeled

3 tablespoons tahini

3 tablespoons hot water

Serves 4

*The roasted red peppers give this humous a tangy sweet taste, which is enhanced by the chilli sauce. This is delicious served with vegetable crudités or spread on wholemeal bread.*

1 Halve the peppers and place under a hot grill for about 20 minutes or until the skins are black. Cover with a clean wet cloth, or place in a plastic bag, and allow to cool for about 10 minutes. Remove the skin from the peppers and blot dry with absorbent kitchen paper.

2 Place the peppers, chickpeas, lemon juice, sweet chilli sauce, olive oil, garlic, tahini and hot water in a food processor or blender and process until smooth. Serve immediately, or cover and chill until needed.

# FALAFEL WITH SALAD IN PITTA

*Chickpeas are a useful source of fibre, B vitamins and minerals. This recipe makes a hearty and nutritious lunch time snack.*

1  Preheat the oven to 180°C, gas mark 4. To make the falafel, mash the chickpeas with the onion and garlic to form a thick pulp. Add the tahini, egg, breadcrumbs, coriander, cumin and salt and mix together well.

2  Divide the falafel mixture into 18 small balls and bake on a baking sheet for 15–20 minutes, or until lightly golden and firm to the touch.

3  To serve, toast the pitta breads, leave to cool slightly and split open. Fill with the shredded lettuce, cherry tomatoes and cucumber. Top the salad with 3 falafel per pitta and drizzle over a little humous, if you like. Sprinkle with a little cayenne pepper or paprika.

## FOR THE FALAFEL

400 g can chickpeas, drained and rinsed

1 red onion, roughly chopped

1 clove garlic, peeled and crushed

3 tablespoons tahini

1 egg, beaten

100 g fresh white breadcrumbs

2 tablespoons fresh coriander, chopped

1 teaspoon ground cumin

½ teaspoon salt

## TO SERVE

6 large pitta breads

Shredded cos lettuce leaves

Cherry tomatoes, halved

½ cucumber, sliced

Humous (see recipe page 34)

Cayenne pepper or paprika, for sprinkling

Serves 6

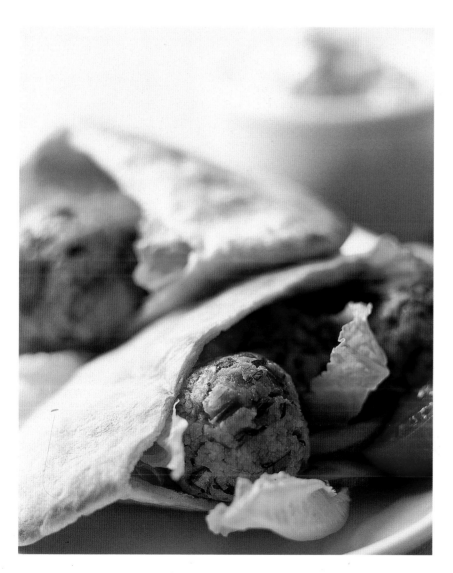

# Quick Ciabatta Pizza

4 ciabatta rolls

3 tablespoons sun-dried tomato paste
or red pesto

1 tablespoon fresh basil leaves, chopped

3 plum tomatoes, thinly sliced

285 g jar artichoke hearts in oil, drained
and roughly chopped

125 g soft rindless goat's cheese,
crumbled

1 tablespoon hazelnuts, chopped

Black pepper, to taste

Olive oil, for drizzling

Fresh basil leaves, to garnish

Serves 4

*A quick and healthy lunch time snack or light supper dish, this can be
served on its own or accompanied by a fresh green salad.*

1   Preheat the oven to 200°C, gas mark 6. Cut the ciabatta rolls in half and
arrange cut-side up on a baking sheet.

2   Spread the sun-dried tomato paste or red pesto over the cut surface of each
toasted roll. Sprinkle over the chopped basil. Place a layer of tomato slices
over the pesto and basil, then top with artichoke hearts and goat's cheese.
Sprinkle over the hazelnuts. Season well with black pepper and drizzle
with a little olive oil.

3   Bake in the oven for about 10 minutes, or until heated through. Garnish
with basil leaves.

# Croque Monsieur

2 slices white or wholemeal bread

15 g butter

1 slice good quality ham

50 g slice Gruyère cheese

Salt and pepper, to taste

2 teaspoons vegetable oil

Serves 1

*This quick snack is great served with a simple mixed salad. If cooking
for two people, double all the ingredients except the oil – if necessary,
use two pans or cook in batches.*

1   Cut the crusts off the bread, then spread one side of each with some of the
butter. Place the ham on the buttered side of one slice of bread, cutting to
fit if necessary, and cover with the Gruyère cheese. Season and top with the
remaining slice of bread, buttered side down.

2   Press the sandwich together firmly, then cut into 4 triangles.

3   Melt the remaining butter with the oil in a non-stick frying pan. Fry the
triangles over a moderate heat, turning once, until golden on both sides.
Press with a fish slice to keep the sandwiches together. Serve hot.

WELSH RAREBIT
Place 50 g grated Cheddar cheese, 15 g butter, 1 tablespoon brown ale,
½ teaspoon mustard and seasoning in a saucepan. Heat very gently, stirring
continuously, until the mixture becomes thick and creamy. Lightly toast one
side of a slice of bread. Pour the sauce over the uncooked side and cook under
a preheated hot grill until it is golden and bubbling. Serve with a crisp green
salad. For buck rarebit, top with a poached egg.

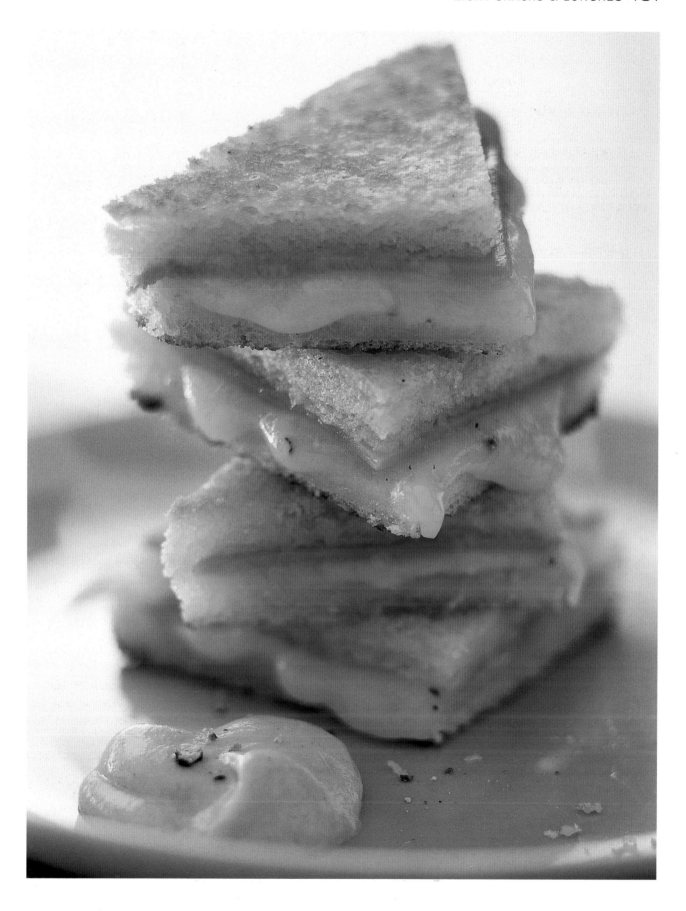

# PEPPERED SMOKED MACKEREL SPREAD

275 g peppered smoked mackerel fillets

200 g soft cheese with herbs and garlic

2 tablespoons fresh flat-leaf parsley, chopped

Zest and juice of 1 lemon

Serves 4

*A quick and easy fish spread made with soft cheese and a hint of lemon. It can be made in advance and frozen, but remember to defrost it thoroughly before serving. Serve with a green salad and toasted Granary bread.*

1   Remove the skin from the smoked mackerel along with any small bones. Flake the fish into a bowl.

2   Add the soft cheese, flat-leaf parsley, lemon zest and juice to the fish and mash together with a fork. Spoon the mixture into a serving bowl. Cover and chill until required.

# CHICKEN TIKKA SALAD

4 tablespoons natural yogurt

4 tablespoons mayonnaise

4 tablespoons grated cucumber

3 spring onions, finely chopped

2 teaspoons fresh mint, chopped

Salt and pepper, to taste

Mixed green salad leaves

450 g ready-made chicken tikka

Sprigs of fresh mint, to garnish

Serves 4

*Mixing the mayonnaise with natural yogurt reduces the fat and boosts the calcium content of this dish. Serve with toasted pitta bread.*

1   Mix the yogurt with the mayonnaise, cucumber, spring onions and mint, blending well to make a dressing. Season to taste. Cover and chill until ready to use.

2   Just before serving, arrange the salad leaves on a large serving plate and top with the chicken tikka. Spoon over the cucumber, mint and yogurt dressing and garnish with sprigs of fresh mint.

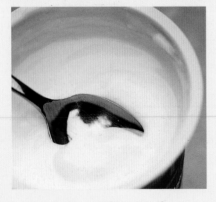

# CHICKEN CAESAR SALAD WITH PARMESAN CRISPS

*The Parmesan crisps in this salad provide plenty of calcium. When serving salads, it is best to put the dressing on at the last moment, as this stops the leaves going soggy.*

1  To make the croutons, cut the bread roughly into small pieces. Heat the olive oil in a large frying pan. Add the bread pieces and cook over a high heat for 3 minutes, stirring occasionally, until crisp and golden. Set aside to cool.

2  Preheat the oven to 200°C, gas mark 6. On a large baking sheet, make 8 heaped piles of grated Parmesan cheese, spacing them well apart. Bake for about 5 minutes until the cheese melts, then remove from the oven and leave to cool.

3  On a chopping board, shred the chicken into bite-sized pieces. Tear the lettuce into pieces and put into a large bowl, then toss in a little of the Caesar salad dressing.

4  Pile the lettuce onto 4 large plates, and top with the chicken. Scatter with the croutons, then drizzle with the remaining Caesar dressing. Break the Parmesan crisps into pieces and sprinkle over the salad. Season with black pepper.

4 slices black olive ciabatta or French bread

2 tablespoons olive oil

8 tablespoons Parmesan cheese, freshly grated

3 cooked chicken breast fillets

Inside leaves of 1 cos lettuce

4–5 tablespoons ready-made Caesar salad dressing

Black pepper, to taste

Serves 4

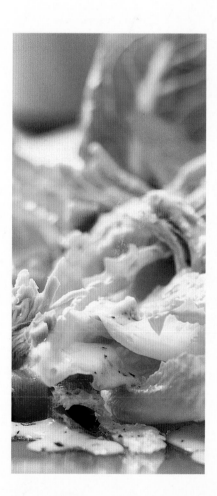

## CAESAR SALAD ON TOASTED CIABATTA
Mix together 1 thinly sliced red onion, 2 shredded spring onions, 4 halved cherry tomatoes, ¼ sliced cucumber and 1 tablespoon extra virgin olive oil. Season well. Preheat the grill to high. Slice a ciabatta lengthways, then cut the 2 pieces in half and toast for 1–2 minutes. Drizzle a little olive oil onto the toasted ciabatta then place 1 cos lettuce leaf on each piece. Fill each leaf with shredded cooked chicken and the salad mixture. Spoon over the Caesar dressing, top with Parmesan shavings and season with black pepper.

## HOME-MADE CAESAR SALAD DRESSING
Put 3 chopped cloves of garlic in a saucepan with 150 ml white wine. Bring to the boil and simmer for 5 minutes. Leave to cool, then put in a food processor or blender with 50 g grated Parmesan cheese, 4 egg yolks, 1 tablespoon Dijon mustard, 2 anchovy fillets and 1 teaspoon white wine vinegar. Blend until well emulsified, then add 300 ml olive oil in a steady stream, until the dressing is smooth. Season well. Store in a jar and keep in the fridge for up to 1 week.

# FETA OMELETTE WITH ROCKET & RED PEPPER

4 large eggs, separated

2 tablespoons fresh mixed herbs, chopped

150 g feta cheese, roughly crumbled

Black pepper, to taste

15 g butter

½ 285 g jar red or mixed peppers in oil, drained and sliced

50 g rocket

Serves 2

*This light and fluffy cheese omelette makes a quick and tasty dish. Serve with a simple plum tomato salad.*

1 Preheat the grill to high. Beat the egg yolks with 3 tablespoons of water, then stir in the herbs, half the feta and plenty of black pepper. In a clean bowl, whisk the egg whites until stiff, then fold into the egg yolk mixture.

2 Over a medium heat, melt the butter in a large non-stick frying pan until foamy, then spoon in the egg mixture. Cook for 3–4 minutes until the underside of the omelette is golden. Remove from the heat and place under the grill for 2–3 minutes, until the top of the omelette is lightly brown.

3 Scatter the pepper slices and the remaining feta evenly over the top of the omelette. Return to the grill and cook for a further 2–3 minutes until the feta begins to melt slightly. Place the rocket evenly over the top of the red pepper and feta and season with black pepper.

4 Fold the omelette in half, then cut in half and serve.

# TWICE-BAKED GOAT'S CHEESE SOUFFLES

40 g butter, plus extra for greasing

25 g Parmesan cheese, freshly grated, plus extra for sprinkling

25 g self-raising flour

225 ml semi-skimmed milk

2 medium eggs, separated

125 g soft rindless goat's cheese, crumbled

Salt and pepper, to taste

Serves 4

*These light and tasty soufflés can be served with a crisp green salad and some wholemeal bread for a healthy lunch time snack. They also make a good first course at a dinner party.*

1 Lightly grease four 150 ml ramekins and sprinkle Parmesan cheese over the base and the sides of the ramekins until evenly coated.

2 Preheat the oven to 180°C, gas mark 4. Melt the butter in a saucepan, then stir in the flour and cook for 1 minute, stirring constantly. Gradually stir in the milk. Bring to the boil and cook for 2–3 minutes, or until the sauce becomes thick and smooth.

3 Allow the sauce to cool slightly then beat in the egg yolks, goat's cheese and seasoning. Whisk the egg whites until they form soft peaks, then, using a metal spoon, carefully fold into the cheese sauce.

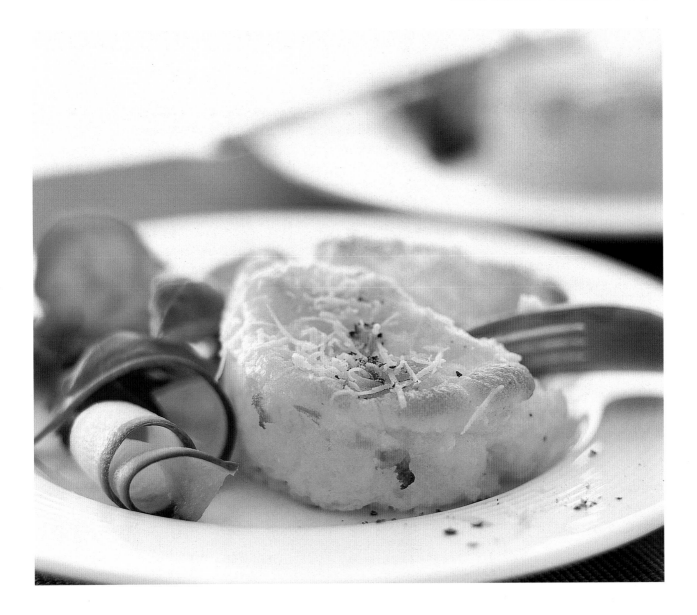

4 Divide the mixture between the ramekins and place in a roasting tin. Pour in enough boiling water to reach halfway up the sides of the ramekins and place in the oven for 20–25 minutes, or until the soufflés are firm to the touch and lightly browned. Remove from the roasting tin and allow to cool. Run a knife around the edge of each soufflé and carefully turn out. Chill until ready to serve.

5 About 30 minutes before serving, heat the oven to 200°C, gas mark 6. Carefully transfer the soufflés to a lightly greased baking sheet, sprinkle with Parmesan cheese and bake for 15–20 minutes or until golden brown.

BLUE CHEESE SOUFFLES
Replace the goat's cheese with Stilton or another blue cheese.

# SPINACH & ROQUEFORT PANCAKES

125 g plain flour, sieved

1 egg, beaten

Pinch of salt

300 ml semi–skimmed milk

Vegetable oil, for frying

500 g fresh spinach, washed

225 g Roquefort or other blue cheese, chopped into small pieces

Serves 4 (makes 8 small pancakes)

*You can use any strong-tasting cheese to make these pancakes, but the combination of salty Roquefort and spinach works particularly well.*

1   Mix the flour, egg and salt together in a large bowl. Gradually beat in enough milk to make a smooth batter with the consistency of single cream.

2   Heat a small pancake pan. When the pan is hot, brush with a little oil and pour in enough batter to thinly coat the base of the pan. Cook over a medium heat for about 1 minute, or until the edges are curling away from the pan and the underside is golden. Using a palette knife, flip the pancake and cook for a further 30 seconds, then turn out onto a sheet of greaseproof paper. Add a little more oil to the pan and repeat the process until all the batter has been used. Cover the pancakes to keep them warm.

3   Place the spinach in a large saucepan with 1 tablespoon of water. Cover and cook until the leaves are just wilted. Transfer to a colander and squeeze out any excess liquid, then chop roughly. Return to the pan and gently reheat.

4   Spoon a little of the spinach into the middle of each of the pancakes and sprinkle over a little of the cheese. Fold the pancakes in half to serve.

# CAJUN CHEESE POTATO SKINS WITH TOMATO & RED ONION SALAD

FOR THE POTATO SKINS

4 baking potatoes

Oil, for brushing

2 tablespoons Cajun seasoning mix

8 thin slices of Cheddar cheese, cut in half

*These are guaranteed to be a big hit with the whole family. Served with a salad, they are ideal for a light lunch, or with grilled chicken or fish for a more substantial meal.*

1   Preheat the oven to 200°C, gas mark 6. Push a metal skewer through each potato (this speeds up the cooking process by about 20 minutes) and bake for 1 hour or until tender.

2   Remove the potatoes from the oven and set aside to cool slightly. Turn the oven up to 225°C, gas mark 7. Remove the skewers and carefully cut each potato into 6 wedges.

3   Brush each potato wedge with a little oil, then dust on both sides with the Cajun seasoning. Put the wedges on a baking sheet and return to the oven for a further 15–20 minutes, until crispy and golden.

4   Meanwhile, make the salad. Slice the tomatoes thinly and place in a shallow dish with the garlic and onion. Whisk the red wine vinegar and

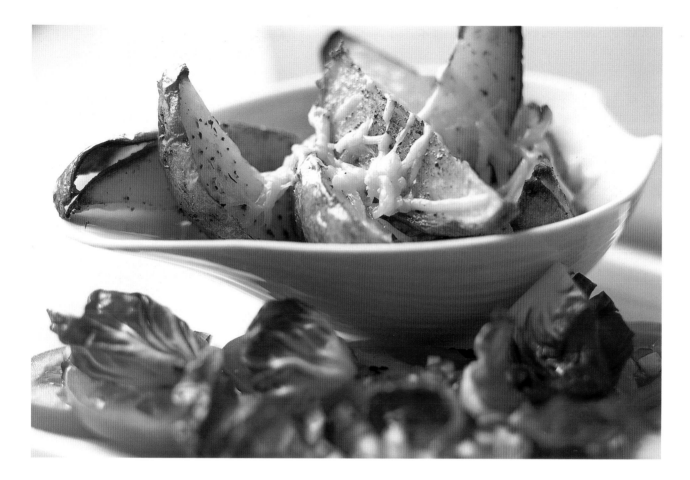

olive oil together, season to taste, then drizzle over the tomato salad. Set aside. Break the radicchio into small pieces, cover and set aside.

5  Remove the potato wedges from the oven and turn the oven off. Arrange the slices of cheese over the wedges and return to the warm oven for 3–4 minutes, or until the cheese has melted.

6  Divide the potato wedges between 4 serving plates with a large spoonful of the tomato and red onion salad and a large handful of the radicchio. Season with a grinding of pepper before serving.

HOME-MADE CAJUN SEASONING
If preferred, you can make your own Cajun seasoning. In a pestle and mortar, pound together 2 tablespoons ground paprika, 2 tablespoons cayenne pepper, 1 tablespoon black pepper, 2 tablespoons garlic granules, 2 tablespoons onion flakes, 1 tablespoon dried oregano, 1 tablespoon dried thyme and 1 tablespoon salt, until you have a powdery consistency. This seasoning can be stored in an airtight jar for up to 3 months.

FOR THE SALAD

4 plum tomatoes

2 cloves garlic, peeled and finely chopped

1 red onion, finely chopped

1 tablespoon red wine vinegar

4 tablespoons extra virgin olive oil

Salt and pepper, to taste

1 head radicchio

Serves 4

# BACON & RICOTTA TART

175 g strong plain four, sieved, plus extra for dusting

1 level teaspoon easy-blend dried yeast

1 level teaspoon salt

½ teaspoon sugar

1 tablespoon olive oil

200 g ricotta cheese

150 ml soured cream

1 medium white onion, thinly sliced

Salt and pepper, to taste

8 rashers lean smoked bacon, roughly chopped

Olive oil, for drizzling

Serves 2–4

*This makes a tasty meal when served with a rocket salad. It is also perfect for a packed lunch or picnic. If time is short, you could use a ready-made pizza base.*

1 To make the dough, place the flour, yeast, salt and sugar in a warm bowl. Mix in the olive oil with 125 ml hand-hot water to make a soft dough. Knead the dough on a floured work surface for 3–4 minutes. Return the dough to the bowl, cover with clingfilm and leave in a warm place to rise for about 1 hour.

2 Meanwhile, to make the topping, mix the ricotta cheese, soured cream and onion together. Add a little salt and plenty of pepper. Preheat the oven to 230°C, gas mark 8 and preheat a baking tray.

3 Once the dough has doubled in size, turn out on to a floured surface. Knead the dough for a couple of minutes to "knock out" the air. Shape the dough into a circle about 25 cm in diameter.

4 Place the dough on the baking tray, spoon over the ricotta mixture, scatter over the bacon and drizzle with olive oil. Cook for 20 minutes or until the bacon is crisp.

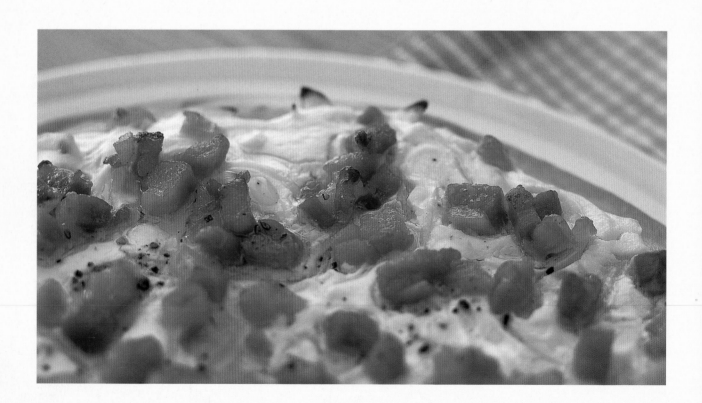

# SWEET POTATO WITH COTTAGE CHEESE & CRISPY BACON

*Although it's low in fat, cottage cheese still provides useful amounts of calcium. Adding a little crispy bacon helps to perk up its flavour.*

1  Preheat the oven to 200°C, gas mark 6. Pierce the potato in several places and wrap in foil. Bake in the oven for 45–60 minutes, or until soft.

2  Cook the bacon under a hot grill until crispy. Chop into small pieces and mix into the cottage cheese.

3  Remove the potato from the foil and slice in half. Spoon over the cottage cheese and bacon mixture and serve.

1 medium sweet potato, about 250 g

2 rashers lean smoked bacon

100 g cottage cheese

Serves 1

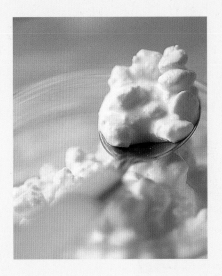

# SPINACH & POTATO CAKE

*Served with a simple tomato salad, this dish makes a healthy and satisfying lunch on a cold day.*

1  Preheat the oven to 180°C, gas mark 4. Melt the butter in a large saucepan, add the garlic and spinach and cook until the spinach is just wilted. Drain well and chop roughly.

2  Mix together the spinach, eggs, crème fraîche, milk, 75 g of the Gruyère cheese and the herbs. Season with salt, pepper and nutmeg.

3  Lightly grease a 23 cm springform cake tin. Cover the base with a layer of sliced potatoes, then a layer of the spinach mixture. Continue layering, finishing with layer of potatoes. Sprinkle with the remaining Gruyère cheese and cover the tin with lightly greased foil. Place in a roasting tin and pour in enough boiling water to reach halfway up the sides of the cake tin.

4  Bake for 1½ hours until the potatoes are tender – remove the foil for the last 15 minutes to allow the top to brown. Allow to cool in the tin for 5–10 minutes before serving.

15 g butter, plus extra for greasing

1 clove garlic, peeled and finely chopped

500 g fresh spinach, washed

3 eggs, beaten

2 x 200 ml cartons reduced-fat crème fraîche

2 tablespoons semi-skimmed milk

125 g Gruyère cheese, grated

3 tablespoons fresh mixed herbs, chopped

Salt and pepper, to taste

Pinch freshly grated nutmeg

4 large potatoes, peeled and thinly sliced

Serves 6

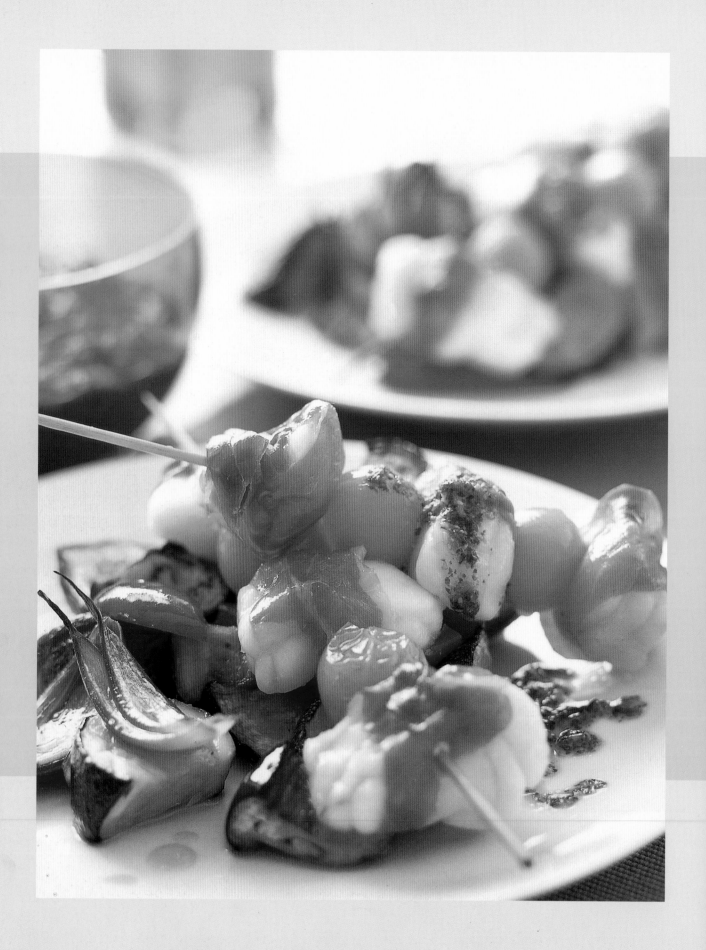

# 4 Main Courses

This chapter features meat, fish and vegetarian main courses, ranging from those suitable for a quick family meal to ideas for a more elaborate dinner party. Most importantly, all the dishes provide essential vitamins and minerals for strong, healthy bones.

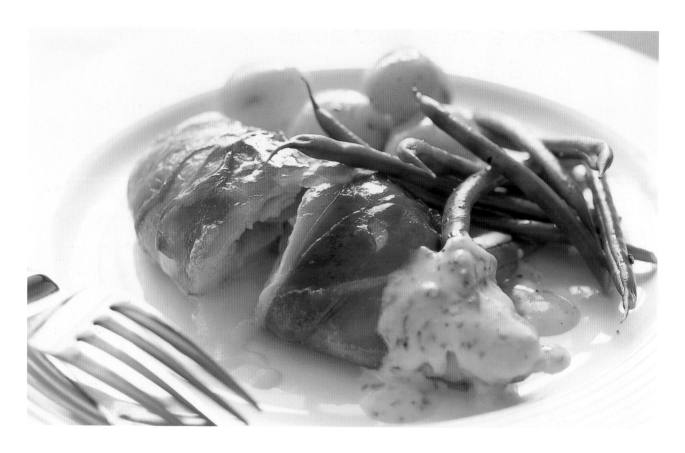

# BRIE-STUFFED CHICKEN WITH CREAMY PESTO

4 boneless, skinless chicken breasts

200 g Brie

8 slices Parma ham

Vegetable oil, for frying

2 tablespoons green pesto

2 tablespoons Greek yogurt

Serves 4

*Mixing Greek yogurt into the pesto gives it a wonderfully creamy flavour and helps to boost the calcium content of this dish. Serve with lightly steamed vegetables and new potatoes.*

1   Cut sideways into each chicken breast to create a pocket. Cut the Brie into 4 slices and stuff one into each piece of chicken. Wrap 2 slices of Parma ham around each piece and secure with cocktail sticks.

2   Place the chicken on a lightly oiled baking tray and cook in the oven at 190°C, gas mark 5 for 35 minutes, or until the chicken is cooked through.

3   Remove the cocktail sticks and transfer the chicken to a warm plate. Mix the pesto and yogurt together in a small bowl and drizzle the mixture over the cooked chicken.

FRESH PESTO
Place 50 g fresh basil, 2 crushed cloves garlic, 2 tablespoons pine nuts, 125 ml olive oil and 50 g freshly grated Parmesan cheese in a blender or food processor and purée until smooth. The fresh pesto will keep for up to 2 weeks in the fridge.

# CHICKEN & WILD MUSHROOM STROGANOFF

*Packets of fresh wild mushrooms can be found in supermarkets, but, if not, you can simply double the amount of chestnut mushrooms. Serve with plain boiled rice or boiled new potatoes.*

1 Cut the chicken into thin strips. Heat the butter and oil in a large deep non-stick frying pan or casserole dish until it foams. Add half the chicken and stir-fry over a high heat for 4–5 minutes until tender and lightly browned. Remove with a slotted spoon and drain on kitchen paper. Set aside. Repeat with the remaining chicken and set aside.

2 Add the onion, mushrooms and red pepper to the frying pan or casserole dish and season well. Sauté over a medium heat for 5 minutes until the onion is soft. Add the tomato purée and cook for 1 minute. Add the stock and sour cream or crème fraîche and stir well. Simmer for about 5 minutes until the mixture thickens slightly.

3 Return the chicken to the dish and simmer for 2–3 minutes to heat through. To serve, divide between 4 warmed plates and sprinkle with snipped chives.

4 boneless, skinless chicken breasts

25 g butter

1 tablespoon olive oil

2 medium red onions, cut into wedges

125 g mixed wild mushrooms, sliced

125 g chestnut mushrooms, sliced

1 red pepper, deseeded and sliced

Salt and pepper, to taste

2 tablespoons sun-dried tomato purée

240 ml chicken stock

150 ml sour cream or crème fraîche

2 tablespoons fresh chives, snipped

Serves 4

# GARLIC CHICKEN IN YOGURT

*The yogurt and almonds boost the calcium content of this spiced chicken dish. Serve with plain boiled basmati rice.*

1 Mix the chilli flakes, cinnamon, 2 tablespoons olive oil, garlic and curry paste together and season well. In a shallow dish, toss the chicken pieces with the curry paste mixture. Cover and leave for 20 minutes.

2 Heat the remaining oil in a large non-stick frying pan. Stir-fry the chicken for 4–5 minutes until tender and lightly browned.

3 Stir in the ground almonds and yogurt and heat through for 2–3 minutes. Sprinkle over the garam masala and coriander and serve immediately.

1 teaspoon crushed chilli flakes

1 teaspoon ground cinnamon

3 tablespoons olive oil

4 cloves garlic, peeled and finely crushed

2 teaspoons hot curry paste

Salt and pepper, to taste

350 g chicken breast fillets, cut into bite-sized pieces

100 g ground almonds, toasted

340 ml Greek yogurt

1 teaspoon garam masala

2 tablespoons fresh coriander, chopped

Serves 4

# CORONATION CHICKEN SALAD

## FOR THE CHICKEN

50 g butter

1 medium onion, finely chopped

8 ready-to-eat dried apricots, finely chopped

Small pinch saffron strands

Zest of 1 lemon

2 tablespoons runny honey

2 tablespoons hot curry paste

200 ml dry white wine

8 tablespoons mayonnaise

8 tablespoons Greek yogurt

450 g skinless, boneless cooked chicken, cut into bite-sized pieces

2 tablespoons fresh coriander, chopped

Salt and pepper, to taste

## FOR THE SALAD

1 red pepper, thinly sliced

1 red chilli, deseeded and thinly sliced

4 spring onions, cut into thin strips

50 g unsalted peanuts, chopped

Wild rocket, to garnish

Fresh coriander sprigs, to garnish

Serves 4–6

*Originally created for the Queen's coronation by the Cordon Bleu Cookery School, this is a more contemporary version. It is ideal for using up left-over cooked chicken, and makes a great sandwich filling.*

1 Melt the butter in a saucepan and cook the onion for 5 minutes until soft. Add the apricots, saffron, lemon zest, honey, curry paste and wine. Simmer uncovered for 25 minutes or until the mixture is the consistency of thin chutney. Leave to cool.

2 Mix the mayonnaise with the yogurt, add the chicken and the cooled curry mixture and mix well. Add the coriander and season to taste.

3 To make the salad, mix together the pepper, chilli, spring onions and peanuts. Divide the chicken between 4–6 plates and top with the salad mixture. Serve with rocket leaves and more coriander.

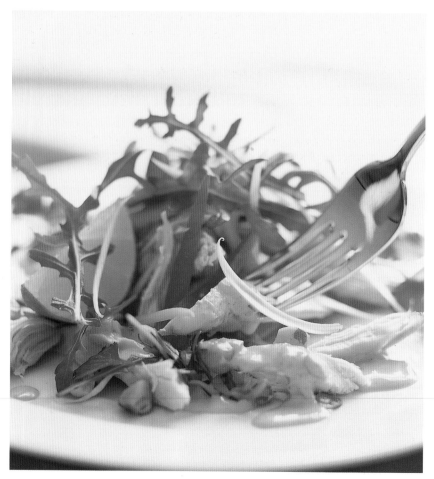

# CHICKEN & SESAME BITES

*Everyone will love these tasty little chicken bites. Sesame seeds have a deliciously nutty flavour and are a useful source of calcium, particularly for people who don't eat dairy products. Serve with a spicy tomato salsa.*

1   Mix together the breadcrumbs, sesame seeds and seasoning, then spread over a large plate or baking tray.

2   Dip the chicken pieces into the beaten egg then roll in the breadcrumb and sesame seed mixture until thoroughly coated. Carefully lay the chicken on a lightly greased baking sheet and place in the fridge for 30 minutes.

3   Meanwhile, preheat the oven to 200°C, gas mark 6. Spray the chicken with olive oil and bake for 10–15 minutes, until the breadcrumbs are golden brown and the chicken cooked through.

75 g fine white breadcrumbs

75 g sesame seeds

Salt and pepper, to taste

2 large skinless chicken breasts, cut into bite-sized pieces

1 egg, beaten

Extra virgin olive oil spray

Serves 4

# QUICK TURKEY CASSOULET

*This is a hearty and wholesome supper dish guaranteed to warm you up on a cold day. Turkey is a useful source of zinc, which is helpful in building strong bones. Serve with a crisp green salad.*

1   Heat 2 tablespoons of the oil in a large non-stick saucepan. Add the onion, garlic, bacon and celery and cook over a low heat for 10 minutes, stirring occasionally.

2   Add the tomatoes, chicken stock and soy sauce. Bring to the boil, then reduce to a fast simmer and cook for about 15 minutes, or until the sauce begins to thicken.

3   Add the mustard, beans and turkey and continue to cook for a further 5 minutes. Transfer the mixture into a shallow ovenproof dish.

4   Mix the breadcrumbs, Parmesan cheese and parsley together and sprinkle over the turkey mixture. Drizzle with the remaining tablespoon of olive oil and place under a medium–hot grill for 5 minutes, or until the breadcrumbs are golden brown.

3 tablespoons olive oil

1 medium red onion, finely chopped

2 cloves garlic, crushed or finely chopped

125 g smoked back bacon, roughly chopped

2 sticks celery, finely chopped

400 g can chopped tomatoes

250 ml chicken stock

2 tablespoons dark soy sauce

2 teaspoons Dijon mustard

2 x 400 g cans mixed beans, rinsed and drained

400 g cooked turkey, roughly chopped

75 g fresh white breadcrumbs

50 g Parmesan cheese, freshly grated

3 tablespoons parsley, chopped

Serves 4

# PORK STUFFED WITH APRICOTS & PINE NUTS

### FOR THE STUFFING

1 tablespoon olive oil

1 medium onion, peeled and finely chopped

40 g fresh white breadcrumbs

40 g ready-to-eat dried apricots, roughly chopped

25 g pine nuts, lightly toasted

2 tablespoons fresh parsley, chopped

Salt and pepper, to taste

1 small egg, beaten

### FOR THE PORK

1 pork loin, about 900 g, trimmed

1 tablespoon olive oil

100 ml white wine

### FOR THE GRAVY

2 teaspoons plain flour

400 ml chicken stock

3 tablespoons Greek yogurt

1 tablespoon wholegrain mustard

Salt and pepper, to taste

Serves 4–6

*Apricots are rich in potassium, which is beneficial for strong bones. They also provide useful amounts of calcium. Serve this for Sunday lunch with potatoes and green vegetables.*

1 Preheat the oven to 180°C, gas mark 4. To make the stuffing, heat the olive oil in a non-stick pan and fry the onion for 4–5 minutes until soft. In a large bowl, mix together the breadcrumbs, apricots, pine nuts, parsley and seasoning. Add the cooked onion and the egg and mix well.

2 Split the pork almost in half, down the length of the loin, and spread the stuffing in the middle. Bring the two cut edges of pork together to enclose the stuffing and tie at intervals with string. Heat the oil in a pan, wait until it is hot, then add the pork and brown on all sides. Transfer the pork to a roasting tin, cut side down. Pour over the wine and cook in the oven for 1 hour. Test that the pork is cooked by piercing the thickest part with a fine skewer – the juices should run clear. Transfer to a warm plate, cover with foil and keep warm while you make the gravy.

3 Put the roasting tin on the hob and stir the flour into the juices from the meat. Gradually stir in the stock and simmer for 5 minutes, until the gravy begins to thicken. Stir in the yogurt and mustard and season to taste. Slice the pork and serve with the gravy.

---

### PORK STUFFED WITH APPLE & WALNUTS

For an alternative stuffing, you can replace the apricots with 40 g dried apple and the pine nuts with 25 g roughly chopped walnuts. To make the gravy use 200 ml chicken stock and 200 ml dry cider.

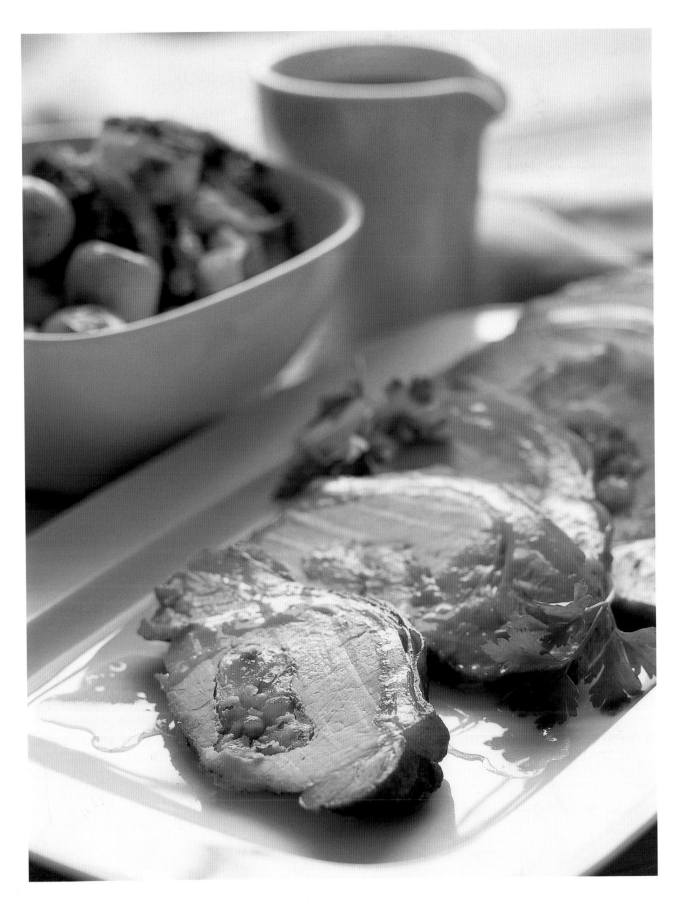

# PORK WITH PAK CHOI & BLACK BEAN SAUCE

2 tablespoons vegetable oil

450 g pork tenderloin, thinly sliced

2 cloves garlic, crushed or finely chopped

2.5 cm fresh ginger, finely chopped

8 spring onions, cut into 0.5 cm slices

125 g shiitake mushrooms

200 g broccoli florets

125 g baby sweetcorn, sliced lengthways

190 g black bean sauce

1 tablespoon runny honey

150 g pak choi, trimmed and sliced

200 g egg noodles

1 tablespoon sesame oil

Spring onions, thinly sliced, to garnish

Serves 4

*Pak choi has a mild and pleasant flavour and a crisp texture. If you can't find pak choi, you can use Chinese cabbage instead.*

1  Heat 1 tablespoon of the vegetable oil in a wok or large frying pan. Add the pork and stir-fry over a high heat for 5 minutes, or until browned. Remove from the pan and set aside.

2  Wipe the wok clean with kitchen paper and heat the remaining vegetable oil. Once the oil is hot, add the garlic, ginger and spring onions and stir-fry for 1 minute. Add the mushrooms, broccoli and sweetcorn and continue cooking for 2–3 minutes.

3  Return the pork to the wok, stir in the black bean sauce, honey, pak choi and 150 ml water. Cook for a further 5 minutes or until the sauce is hot.

4  Meanwhile, cook the noodles according to the manufacturer's instructions. Drain well, then stir through the sesame oil. To serve, place the noodles and pork stir-fry in a bowl and garnish with spring onions.

# PORK ESCALOPES WITH CELERIAC CREAM MASH

### FOR THE MASH

450 g celeriac, peeled and cut into even-sized pieces

450 g potatoes, peeled and cut into even-sized pieces

Small knob butter

3 spring onions, finely chopped

150 ml crème fraîche

Salt and pepper, to taste

*The dense texture of celeriac makes a delicious creamy mash, which provides an excellent accompaniment to plain meats, such as pork.*

1  Bring a large pan of salted water to the boil. Add the celeriac and potato, bring back to the boil and cook for 20–30 minutes, or until both are tender. Drain well, return to the pan and mash.

2  In a small pan, heat the butter and cook the spring onions for 2–3 minutes, until soft. Add the crème fraîche and warm through for 1 minute. Add the mixture to the mash, beat well and season. Cover and keep warm until ready to serve.

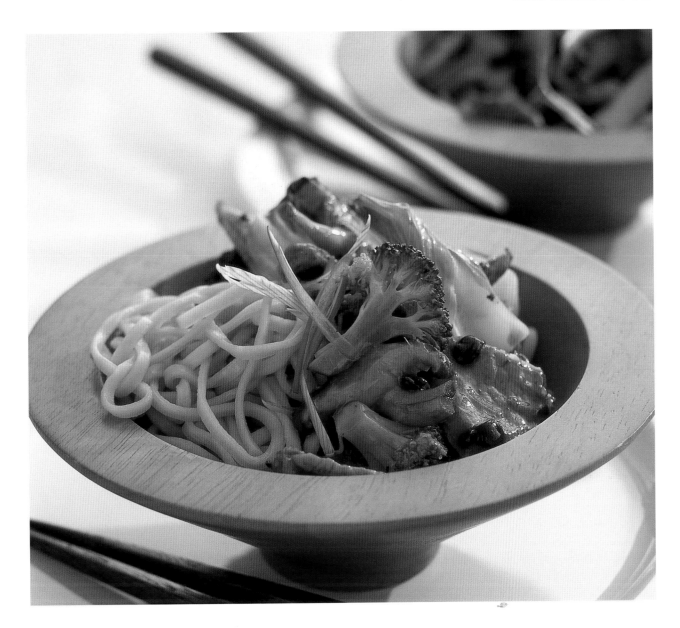

3  Meanwhile, put the escalopes between two sheets of greaseproof paper and thin by beating with a rolling pin. Brush each escalope with the melted butter and coat both sides with the breadcrumbs.

4  Heat the grill to medium. Arrange the breaded escalopes on a foil-lined grill rack and grill for 3–4 minutes on each side.

5  Serve the escalopes on warm serving plates with a large spoonful of the celeriac mash. Garnish with sage leaves and freshly ground black pepper.

### FOR THE ESCALOPES

4 pork escalopes, each about 125 g

25 g butter, melted

50 g fine white breadcrumbs

Fresh sage leaves, to garnish

Freshly ground black pepper

Serves 4

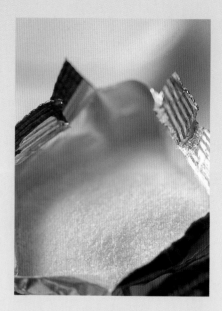

# POLENTA WITH BACON & MUSHROOMS

*Polenta, which is made from cornmeal, is a speciality of northern Italy. For a change, you could replace the Parmesan with a blue cheese, such as Stilton, or goat's cheese.*

1 Place 700 ml of salted water in a large non-stick saucepan and bring to the boil. Pour in the polenta in a slow steady stream, stirring continuously. Reduce the heat and cook for 1 minute, or until the polenta is thick. Remove from the heat, stir in the Parmesan cheese, herbs and butter and more salt, if required.

2 Spread the polenta into a shallow lightly oiled tin, to a thickness of about 1 cm. Allow to cool, then cut into triangles.

3 Heat the oil in a large non-stick frying pan. Add the bacon and cook over a high heat for 5 minutes, until it begins to brown. Add the spring onions and mushrooms and continue to cook for a further 5 minutes. Add the stock, season to taste and reduce the heat slightly. Cook for 20–30 minutes or until the liquid has reduced. Stir in the yogurt.

4 Place the polenta triangles under a preheated grill for 3–4 minutes, turn and continue to cook for a further 3 minutes. Transfer to warm plates, spoon over the bacon and mushroom mixture and serve.

175 g quick-cook polenta

125 g Parmesan cheese, freshly grated

3 tablespoons fresh mixed herbs, roughly chopped

15 g butter

Salt, to taste

1 tablespoon olive oil

225 g rindless smoked back bacon, roughly chopped

8 spring onions, chopped

300 g mixed mushrooms, roughly chopped

300 ml chicken stock

Salt and pepper, to taste

6 tablespoons Greek yogurt

Serves 4

MUSHROOM POLENTA
This recipe can be adapted for vegetarians by simply omitting the bacon and using vegetable stock instead of chicken stock.

# Broccoli & Smoked Ham Tagliatelle

*If you do not have fresh pasta, dried pasta can also be used in this dish – pasta shells work particularly well. Serve with a crisp green salad.*

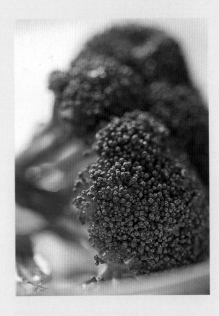

1  Cook the pasta in boiling salted water for 3–4 minutes, according to the packet instructions, until *al dente*.

2  Meanwhile, melt the butter in a large saucepan, add the onion, broccoli and yellow pepper and fry for 5–7 minutes until just softened. Stir in the mascarpone cheese and heat through for 1–2 minutes until soft. Add the smoked ham, grated nutmeg and flat-leaf parsley.

3  Fold the pasta into the sauce, season to taste and heat through for 1–2 minutes. Heat the grill to high. Turn the pasta into a shallow heatproof dish, sprinkle with Cheddar cheese and grill until golden and bubbling.

---

VEGETABLE TAGLIATELLE

For a delicious vegetarian alternative, omit the ham and replace with 225 g mixture of any vegetables that can be cooked quickly, such as mange tout, mushrooms or leeks.

225 g fresh green or white tagliatelle

25 g butter

1 large onion, halved and sliced

225 g small broccoli florets

1 yellow pepper, deseeded and chopped

250 g mascarpone cheese

225 g smoked ham, shredded

½ teaspoon grated nutmeg

2 tablespoons flat-leaf parsley, chopped

Salt and pepper, to taste

125 g Cheddar cheese, grated

Serves 4

# SKEWERED LAMB WITH TOMATO, CHILLI & YOGURT MARINADE

### FOR THE LAMB

700 g lamb neck fillet, trimmed and cut into chunks

1 tablespoon olive oil

2 cloves garlic, crushed

3 small red chillies, deseeded and finely chopped

25 g sun-dried tomatoes in oil, drained and finely chopped

2 teaspoons balsamic vinegar

Pinch soft brown sugar

100 ml natural yogurt

Freshly ground black pepper, to taste

*These tender marinated chunks of lamb are delicious served with basmati rice. Look out for small jars of chopped chillies in sunflower oil, as this speeds up the preparation and avoids the need to handle fresh chillies, which can be off-putting for some people.*

1 Place the lamb, oil, garlic, chillies, sun-dried tomatoes, balsamic vinegar, brown sugar and yogurt together in a shallow bowl and stir well. Season with freshly ground black pepper. Cover, place in the fridge and leave to marinate for at least 3 hours, or preferably overnight. Soak 4 wooden skewers in cold water for 30 minutes before using.

2 To make the rice, bring a large pan of water to the boil, stir in the rice and add a pinch of salt. Return to the boil, cover and simmer for 12–14 minutes, or cook according to the manufacturer's instructions. Drain well. Stir in the chopped coriander and sun-dried tomatoes.

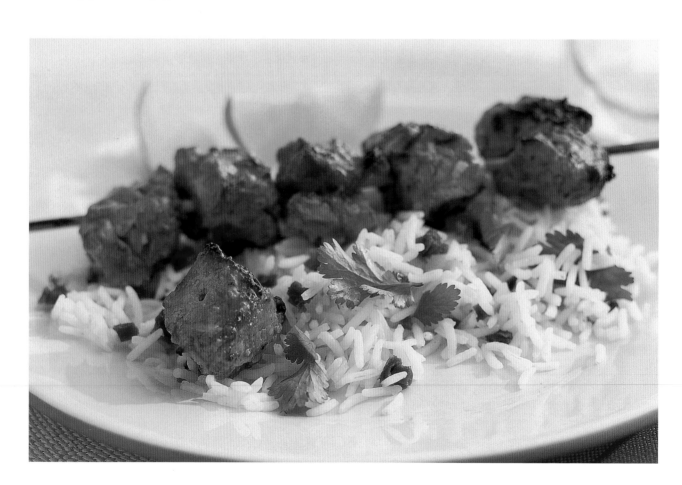

3  Heat the grill to high. Thread the lamb onto the skewers, reserving the marinade. Put the skewered lamb on a grill rack and grill for 3–4 minutes on each side for rare, or 5–6 minutes on each side for well done. Brush with the reserved marinade during grilling.

4  Serve the lamb on the skewers with the rice. Garnish with lime wedges and coriander sprigs.

## GARLIC & CUMIN ROASTED LAMB WITH APRICOT & CHICKPEA SALSA

*Here, roast lamb is given an unusual twist when served with a tangy salsa. The salsa can be made in advance and stored, covered, in the fridge until ready to serve – remove from the fridge while cooking the lamb to allow the flavours to develop.*

1  Preheat the oven to 200°C, gas mark 6. Rub the cumin seeds over the lamb fillets. Using a small sharp knife, make small cuts all over the fillets and insert the garlic slivers.

2  Put the lamb fillets into a roasting tin and roast in the oven for 30 minutes, until tender.

3  Meanwhile, make the salsa. Combine the red onion, chilli, sun-dried tomatoes, apricots, chickpeas, oil, lime zest and juice and coriander together in a bowl. Cover and set aside.

4  When the lamb is cooked, remove from the oven and leave to stand for 5 minutes. To serve, slice the lamb and top with the salsa. Garnish with mint leaves.

### FOR THE RICE

250 g easy-cook basmati rice

Pinch of salt

2 tablespoons fresh coriander, chopped

1 tablespoon sun-dried tomatoes in oil, drained and finely chopped

Lime wedges, to garnish

Fresh coriander sprigs, to garnish

Serves 4

1 teaspoon cumin seeds

6 lamb neck fillets

2 garlic cloves, cut into slivers

### FOR THE SALSA

1 small red onion, finely chopped

1 red chilli, deseeded and finely chopped

2 sun-dried tomatoes, finely chopped

125 g ready-to-eat dried apricots, finely chopped

300 g canned chickpeas, drained and rinsed

1 tablespoon olive oil

Zest and juice of 1 lime

1 tablespoon fresh coriander, chopped

Mint leaves, to garnish

Serves 4

# MOROCCAN LAMB WITH CHICKPEAS & APRICOTS

2 teaspoons ground ginger

2 teaspoons ground cumin

2 teaspoons paprika

1 cinnamon stick

100 ml orange juice

450 g lamb fillet, cut into bite-sized pieces

1 tablespoon vegetable oil

8 shallots or baby onions, peeled

2 cloves garlic, peeled and crushed

1 tablespoon plain flour

1 tablespoon tomato purée

200 ml chicken stock

150 ml sherry

Salt and pepper, to taste

125 g ready-to-eat dried apricots

400 g can chickpeas, drained and rinsed

Fresh coriander, chopped, to garnish

Serves 4

*Here, the lamb is marinated in a tangy, spicy marinade, which gives it a delicious flavour. Both chickpeas and apricots are good sources of calcium, so this dish is great for people on dairy-free diets. Serve with couscous or plain rice.*

1  Put the ginger, cumin, paprika and the cinnamon stick in a large bowl and pour over the orange juice. Add the lamb and mix well. Cover and leave in a cool place for at least 1 hour, or preferably overnight.

2  Preheat the oven to 180°C, gas mark 4. Heat the oil in a large flameproof casserole dish. Remove the lamb from the marinade and cook it in the dish over a high heat for 5 minutes until lightly browned. Remove with a slotted spoon and set aside.

3  Lower the heat and add a little more oil if necessary. Cook the onions and garlic for 3 minutes, or until they are just beginning to brown. Return the lamb to the dish, stir in the flour and tomato purée and continue cooking for 1 minute, stirring frequently.

4  Add the remaining marinade, stock, sherry and season to taste. Bring to the boil then reduce the heat, cover and bake in the oven for 1 hour.

5  Add the apricots and chickpeas and return to the oven for a further 15 minutes. Garnish with chopped coriander and serve.

MOROCCAN LAMB WITH BUTTER BEANS & PRUNES
For a change, try replacing the chickpeas with canned butter beans and the apricots with prunes.

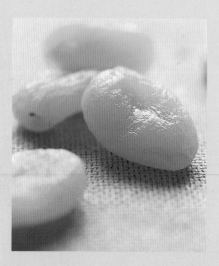

# MOUSSAKA

*The combination of ricotta, Parmesan and Cheddar cheeses makes this warm and comforting dish a real calcium booster. Choose lean minced lamb to help reduce the fat content. Serve with a mixed green salad.*

1 Preheat the oven to 180°C, gas mark 4. Heat 1 tablespoon of the oil in a non-stick saucepan, add the onion and garlic and fry for 5 minutes, or until soft.

2 Add the lamb and cook until tender and browned. Add the tomatoes, tomato purée, cinnamon, oregano and seasoning. Bring to the boil and cook over a low heat for about 20 minutes.

3 Place the potato in a large pan of boiling salted water and cook for 5 minutes. Drain well. Brush the aubergine with the remaining oil and place under a hot grill for 4 minutes on each side, until nicely browned.

4 Mix together the ricotta and Parmesan cheeses. Stir in the beaten egg and milk and season to taste.

5 Arrange half of the grilled aubergine over the base of a shallow ovenproof dish. Spoon over the meat sauce, cover with the remaining aubergine and top with the sliced potatoes.

6 Pour over the cheese sauce, sprinkle with the Cheddar cheese and bake in the oven for 30–40 minutes.

2 tablespoons olive oil

1 large red onion, peeled and finely chopped

2 cloves garlic, crushed or finely chopped

450 g lean minced lamb

2 x 400 g cans chopped tomatoes

1 tablespoon sun-dried tomato purée

¼ teaspoon ground cinnamon

1 teaspoon dried oregano

Salt and pepper, to taste

1 large potato, peeled and thinly sliced

1 large aubergine, cut into slices 0.5 cm thick

250 g ricotta cheese

50 g fresh Parmesan cheese, grated

1 egg, beaten

4 tablespoons full-fat milk

25 g Cheddar cheese, grated

Serves 4

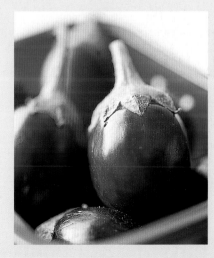

# SHEPHERD'S PIE

450 g minced lamb

1 large onion, chopped

1 bay leaf

50 g mushrooms, sliced

2 medium carrots, sliced

25 g plain flour

300 ml passata

1 tablespoon sun-dried tomato purée

Salt and pepper, to taste

700 g potatoes, peeled and cut into even-sized pieces

25 g butter

4 tablespoons full-fat milk

75 g Lancashire cheese, crumbled

Serves 4

*This version has more flavoursome ingredients than many traditional shepherd's pie recipes and has a delicious cheese topping. Serve with a steamed green vegetable, such as broccoli.*

1  Dry fry the minced lamb with the onion, bay leaf, mushrooms and carrots for 8–10 minutes.

2  Add the flour and cook, stirring, for 1 minute. Gradually blend in the passata and tomato purée. Cook, stirring, until the mixture thickens and boils. Cover and simmer gently for 25 minutes.

3  Remove the bay leaf and season to taste. Spoon into an ovenproof dish.

4  Heat the oven to 200°C, gas mark 6. Cook the potatoes in boiling salted water for 20 minutes, until tender. Drain well and mash with the butter and milk. Spread the mashed potato over the mince mixture and sprinkle with the crumbled cheese. Bake for 15–20 minutes until golden brown.

# BLUE CHEESE & WALNUT STEAKS

125 g Stilton or other blue cheese, crumbled

25 g butter, softened

50–75 g shelled walnut pieces, finely chopped

Freshly ground black pepper, to taste

4 sirloin or fillet steaks, each weighing about 125–180 g, trimmed

Serves 4

*These steaks have a tasty, and unexpectedly crunchy, topping. Simple accompaniments, such as boiled potatoes and a mixed salad, are all that are needed to complete this meal.*

1  Put the cheese in a bowl and mash with a fork. Add butter and walnuts and mix thoroughly. Season to taste with pepper.

2  Preheat the grill to high. Put the steaks on a grill rack and season with plenty of pepper. Place under the grill and cook for 1–2 minutes on each side for rare, 4 minutes on each side for medium and 6–7 minutes on each side for well done.

3  Remove the steaks from under the grill and sprinkle with the cheese and nut mixture. Press down the mixture with a palette knife. Grill for 1 minute, or until the topping is melted and bubbling. Serve immediately.

# MEATBALLS WITH MOZZARELLA & TOMATO SAUCE

*The mozzarella cheese melts while the meatballs are cooking to give a deliciously creamy filling. Combined with a rich tomato sauce, this makes a comforting supper, when served with a large plate of spaghetti.*

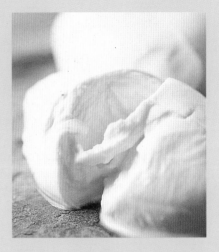

1   To make the meatballs, heat the olive oil in a large non-stick pan. Add the onion and the garlic and cook over a low heat for 5 minutes, until soft. Place the minced beef, breadcrumbs, egg and Parmesan cheese in a bowl. Add the cooked onions and garlic and mix well.

2   Cut or tear the mozzarella cheese into 20 small pieces. Take a heaped tablespoon of the mince mixture and shape into a ball around a piece of mozzarella cheese. Repeat the process with the remaining meat, until you have 20 meatballs. Place the meatballs on a plate or tray and chill for 30 minutes.

3   To make the sauce, heat the oil in a saucepan, add the onion and cook for 4–5 minutes. Add the garlic, tomatoes, tomato purée, mixed herbs, red wine and seasoning. Bring to the boil, reduce the heat, cover and simmer over a low heat for 15 minutes, stirring occasionally. Remove the lid, add the meatballs and continue to cook for a further 20 minutes. Serve the meatballs with the sauce poured over.

## FOR THE MEATBALLS

1 tablespoon olive oil

½ small onion, finely chopped

½ clove garlic, peeled and finely chopped

450 g lean minced beef

50 g fine white breadcrumbs

1 egg, beaten

2 tablespoons Parmesan cheese, freshly grated

75 g mozzarella cheese

## FOR THE SAUCE

1 tablespoon olive oil

½ small onion, finely chopped

½ clove garlic, peeled and finely chopped

2 x 400 g cans chopped tomatoes

1 tablespoon tomato purée

1 teaspoon dried mixed herbs

150 ml red wine

Salt and pepper, to taste

Serves 4

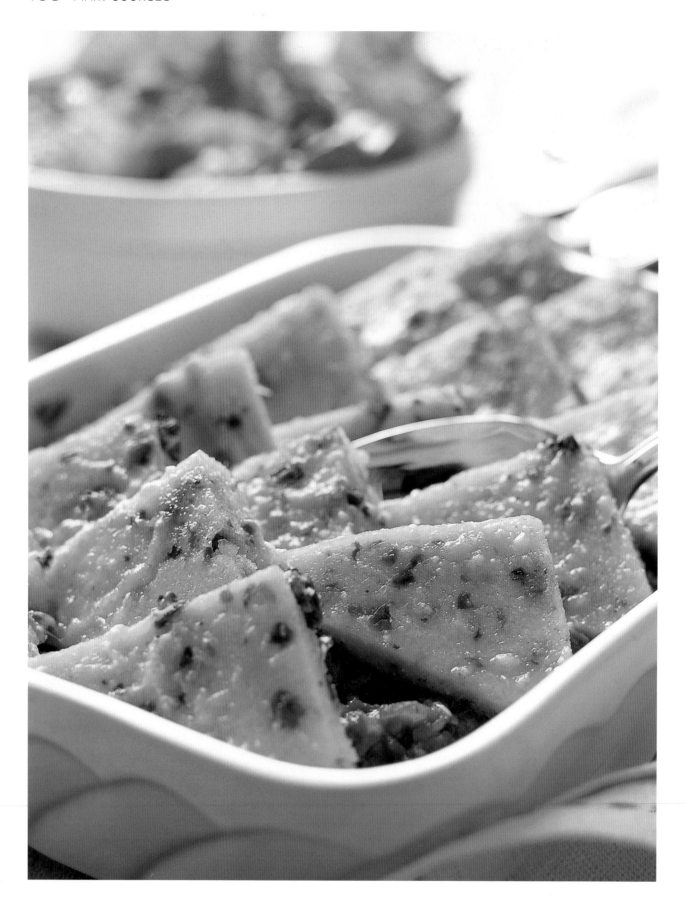

# MINCED BEEF WITH POLENTA TOPPING

*Polenta is gluten-free, so this is a good alternative to a pastry-topped pie for anyone who can't eat wheat or gluten. Mixing Parmesan cheese with the polenta helps boost both the flavour and the calcium content. Serve with a green salad.*

1 Heat the oil in large non-stick saucepan. Add the onion and garlic and cook for 5 minutes until soft. Add the beef and cook until browned.

2 Stir in the tomatoes, tomato paste, wine and seasoning and bring to the boil. Reduce the heat and simmer gently for 30 minutes.

3 To make the polenta topping, place 700 ml of salted water in a large saucepan and bring to the boil. Pour in the polenta in a slow steady stream, stirring continuously. Reduce the heat to low and cook for 1 minute or until the polenta is thick. Stir in the Parmesan cheese, the sun-dried tomatoes, rosemary and butter and add more salt, if required. Spread the polenta into a shallow lightly oiled tin, to a thickness of about 1 cm. Allow to cool.

4 Once the polenta is cold, cut it into triangles. Heat the oven to 200°C, gas mark 6. Place the beef mixture in a shallow ovenproof dish and arrange the polenta over the top so that the triangles overlap slightly.

5 Sprinkle with Parmesan cheese and bake for 20–30 minutes, until the topping is golden brown.

---

OLIVE & STILTON POLENTA TOPPING
Adding different flavours to the polenta topping transforms this recipe. Add 50 g pitted, roughly chopped black olives to the polenta and use 150 g crumbled Stilton or another blue cheese instead of the Parmesan.

1 tablespoon olive oil

1 medium red onion, peeled and finely chopped

1 large clove garlic, finely chopped

450 g lean minced beef

2 x 400 g cans chopped tomatoes

2 tablespoons sun-dried tomato paste

200 ml red wine

Salt and pepper, to taste

## FOR THE POLENTA TOPPING

100 g quick-cook polenta

75 g Parmesan cheese, freshly grated, plus extra for sprinkling

75 g sun-dried tomatoes, roughly chopped

½ teaspoon fresh rosemary, chopped

10 g butter

Salt, to taste

Vegetable oil, for greasing

Serves 4

# SALMON FISH CAKES

550 g floury potatoes, such as Desirée or King Edwards, peeled and cut into large chunks

2 tablespoons mayonnaise

418 g can red salmon, drained

Salt and pepper, to taste

Plain flour, for dusting

1 large egg, beaten

100 g fine white breadcrumbs

4 tablespoons sunflower oil

Lemon wedges, to garnish

Serves 4

*Nutritionists recommend that we eat at least two servings of oil-rich fish, such as salmon, a week. As well as providing healthy omega-3 fatty acids, canned salmon, when eaten with the bones, is an excellent source of calcium. Serve the fish cakes with tzatziki and new potatoes.*

1   Place the potatoes in a large pan of salted water, bring to the boil and cook for about 20 minutes, until tender. Drain well and mash with the mayonnaise.

2   Place the salmon, including the bones, in a large bowl and mash with a fork. Add the mashed potato and season to taste. Mix well, then cover and place in the fridge for 1 hour.

3   Remove the mixture from the fridge. Shape into 8 fish cakes and dust with flour. Carefully dip each fish cake into the beaten egg, then into the breadcrumbs, making sure it is evenly coated.

4   Heat half the oil in a large non-stick frying pan and cook half the fish cakes over a high heat for 4 minutes each side, until the breadcrumbs are golden brown. Drain on absorbent kitchen paper, then transfer to a warm oven while you cook the remaining fish cakes. Garnish with lemon wedges.

# SALMON & LEEK LASAGNE

25 g butter

2 large leeks, washed and thinly sliced

40 g plain flour

600 ml semi-skimmed milk

225 g Cheddar cheese, grated

Salt and pepper, to taste

213 g can pink salmon, drained and flaked

8 sheets fresh lasagne

2 tablespoons sunflower seeds, toasted

Serves 4

*Canned salmon provides a useful source of calcium, vitamin D and phosphorus, all of which are essential for strong bones. Serve this lasagne with a large green salad and crusty bread.*

1   Preheat the oven to 190°C, gas mark 5. Grease a shallow ovenproof dish.

2   Heat the butter in a large non-stick frying pan, add the leeks and cook for 4–5 minutes until soft.

3   Place the flour and milk in a small saucepan, whisk together, then slowly bring to the boil, stirring continuously. Reduce the heat and simmer for 1 minute. Remove from the heat, stir in half of the cheese and season to taste.

4   Mix the leeks, half of the cheese sauce and the salmon together. Spoon half the salmon and leek mixture into the bottom of the prepared dish and top with a layer of fresh lasagne. Spoon over the remaining salmon mixture, top with a final layer of lasagne and pour over the remaining cheese sauce. Sprinkle with the remaining cheese and the sunflower seeds. Bake in the oven for 20 minutes, until the top is bubbling.

# SMOKED SALMON & DILL QUICHE

*The sweet aniseed flavour of the dill complements the smoked salmon perfectly in this nourishing, creamy dish.*

1   Roll out the pastry on a lightly floured surface and use to line a 23 × 4 cm deep, loose-bottomed flan tin. Place on a baking sheet, cover and chill in the fridge for 30 minutes. Preheat the oven to 200°C, gas mark 6.

2   Prick the base of the flan, line with a large sheet of greaseproof paper and fill with baking beans. Bake for 10–15 minutes, then carefully remove the paper and the beans. Return to the oven for a further 5 minutes until the base is firm to the touch and lightly golden. Remove from the oven and set aside while making the filling.

3   Heat the oil and cook the onion for 5 minutes until soft. Turn down the oven to 170°C, gas mark 3. Whisk the eggs and cheeses together until smooth, then whisk in the cream, dill and pepper. Scatter the onion and salmon over the base of the flan case and pour over the egg mixture.

4   Bake the quiche for 45–55 minutes, until lightly set. Garnish with smoked salmon trimmings and dill sprigs.

225 g ready-made shortcrust pastry

Plain flour, for dusting

1 tablespoon oil

1 large onion, finely chopped

2 eggs

200 g full-fat soft cream cheese

25 g rindless soft goat's cheese

300 ml single cream

1 tablespoon fresh dill, chopped, plus extra to garnish

Pepper, to taste

125 g smoked salmon trimmings, roughly chopped, plus extra to garnish

Serves 6

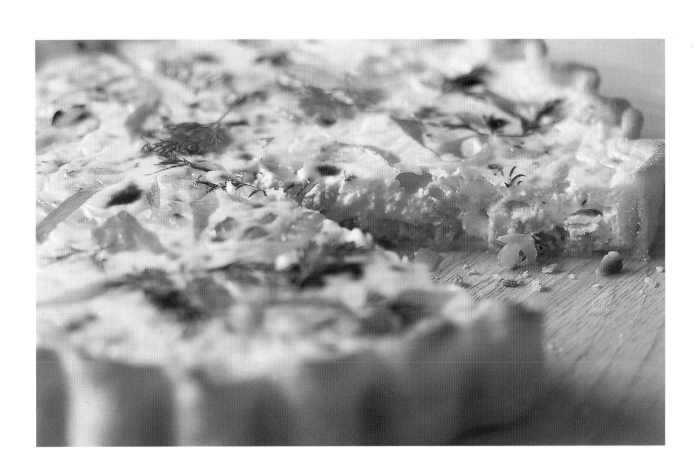

# QUICK SALMON KEDGEREE

225 g basmati rice

2 teaspoons olive oil

4 spring onions, roughly chopped

213 g can salmon, drained, bones and skin removed, then roughly flaked

½ teaspoon coriander seeds, finely crushed

3 tablespoons double cream

3 hard-boiled eggs, quartered

3 tablespoons fresh flat-leaf parsley, chopped, plus extra to garnish

Salt and pepper, to taste

2 lemons, cut into wedges, to garnish

Serves 4

*Oil-rich fish, such as salmon, are one of the few dietary sources of vitamin D, which is essential for the absorption of calcium. This delicious rice dish is ideal for brunch.*

1  Bring a large pan of salted water to the boil. Stir in the rice and return to the boil, then cover and simmer for 12–14 minutes until just tender. Drain the rice well, rinse with boiling water and drain again.

2  Meanwhile, heat the oil in a large non-stick frying pan and cook the spring onions for 1–2 minutes until soft.

3  Add the cooked rice, salmon, coriander seeds, cream, hard-boiled eggs and chopped parsley. Season lightly and heat through gently for 2 minutes.

4  Spoon the kedgeree onto warmed serving plates and garnish with the lemon wedges, flat-leaf parsley sprigs and a grinding of black pepper.

TUNA KEDGEREE

This kedgeree can also be made with tuna. Replace the salmon with 213 g canned tuna in sunflower oil – drain and flake the tuna before using.

# SALMON WITH A CRUMB CRUST

50 g fine white breadcrumbs

1 tablespoon pine nuts, lightly toasted

4 tablespoons fresh basil, chopped

15 g butter

50 g Parmesan cheese, freshly grated

Salt and pepper, to taste

4 salmon fillets

Serves 4

*This recipe is quick and easy and is an ideal dish for a quick midweek supper party – serve with new potatoes and green beans.*

1  Heat the grill. Place the breadcrumbs, pine nuts, basil, butter, Parmesan cheese and seasoning in a food processor and blend until combined.

2  Place the salmon under a moderately hot grill for 5 minutes. Turn over, top with the breadcrumb mixture, pressing it down gently with the palm of your hand. Grill for a further 5 minutes, or until the salmon is cooked through.

# COD & BROCCOLI CHEESE PIE

*Here, chunks of fish are cooked in a creamy cheese sauce, under a layer*
*of golden cheese and mashed potato. Mascarpone cheese is a quick way*
*to make a cheese sauce and is a good source of calcium.*

1 Preheat the oven to 180°C, gas mark 4. Place the cod in an ovenproof dish
and pour over 450 ml of the milk. Add the onion, carrot and the bay
leaf. Cover and cook in the oven for 20 minutes. Strain off, and discard,
the milk.

2 Meanwhile, cook the potatoes in boiling water for 20 minutes. Drain and
return to the saucepan. Add 25 g of the butter and mash smoothly. Add the
cream and the remaining milk and beat until light and fluffy. Season well,
then fold in half the Cheddar cheese.

3 In the meantime, blanch the broccoli in boiling salted water for 1 minute.
Drain well and rinse under cold running water. Set aside on a plate lined
with kitchen paper.

4 Melt 25 g of the butter in a saucepan and cook the leeks for 5–7 minutes,
until softened. Add the mascarpone and stir well until smooth. Cook for
5–7 minutes until thickened. Stir the chopped dill into the mascarpone and
season well.

5 Turn the oven up to 230°C, gas mark 8. Flake the cod in the ovenproof dish,
place the broccoli evenly over the flaked fish, then pour over the sauce.
Spoon over the mashed potato, covering the filling completely, and
sprinkle over the remaining Cheddar cheese. Dot with the remaining butter
and bake in the oven for 10–15 minutes until brown on top. Serve
garnished with sprigs of fresh dill.

---

### SALMON & BROCCOLI CHEESE PIE
Replace the fresh cod with 750 g fresh salmon fillet. Flavour the mashed
potato with some finely chopped spring onions or chopped fresh herbs, such
as dill, tarragon or chervil.

---

### PARSNIP TOPPING
Replace half of the potatoes with parsnips to make a parsnip mash topping,
then follow the recipe as above.

---

### CARROT TOPPING
For a potato and carrot topping, use 750 g potato and fold 225 g grated carrot
into the mash, then follow the recipe as above.

---

750 g cod fillet

600 ml full-fat milk

½ onion, sliced

1 carrot, thinly sliced

1 bay leaf

1 kg floury potatoes, such as Maris Piper,
peeled and cut into even-sized pieces

75 g butter

150 ml single cream

Salt and pepper, to taste

100 g mature Cheddar cheese, grated

225 g small broccoli florets

1 large leek, thinly sliced

500 g mascarpone cheese

1 tablespoon fresh dill, chopped, plus
extra to garnish

Serves 6

# COD BAKED IN YOGURT

150 ml natural yogurt

1 clove garlic, peeled and finely chopped

2.5 cm piece fresh root ginger, peeled and finely chopped

½ teaspoon ground cumin

½ teaspoon ground coriander

¼ teaspoon chilli powder

¼ teaspoon salt

4 skinless cod fillets

Serves 4

*This dish is low in fat, making it a good choice for anyone on a weight-reducing or low-fat diet. If you haven't got the individual spices to hand, you could use 1 tablespoon of curry paste instead. Serve the fish with a tomato salad and naan bread.*

1  Mix together the yogurt, garlic, ginger, cumin, coriander, chilli and salt.

2  Place the fish in a shallow dish and pour over the spiced yogurt mixture. Cover and refrigerate for 2–3 hours.

3  Heat the grill. Transfer the fish onto a foil-lined grill pan and cook under a hot grill for 5–8 minutes, or until the fish is cooked through.

# POACHED HADDOCK WITH SPINACH & POACHED EGG

2 smoked haddock fillets, about 150 g each

150 ml full-fat milk

2 large eggs

225 g baby spinach leaves, washed and drained

Salt and pepper, to taste

Serves 2

*This dish makes a healthy and nutritious lunch or light supper. Spinach provides useful amounts of calcium, particularly for people who don't eat dairy products. Egg yolks are rich in vitamin K which is essential for bone health.*

1  Place the haddock in a large shallow pan and pour over the milk. Cover and simmer gently for about 8 minutes, or until cooked through.

2  Meanwhile, bring a pan of water to the boil, then carefully crack the eggs into the water and poach for 2–3 minutes. Remove with a slotted spoon, allowing the water to drain thoroughly. Set aside on plate lined with kitchen paper.

3  Cook the spinach in a large saucepan for 2–3 minutes until just wilted – there is no need to add extra water as enough clings to the leaves after washing. Drain, and season well.

4  Divide the spinach between two plates and place a fillet of haddock upon each. Top each with a poached egg.

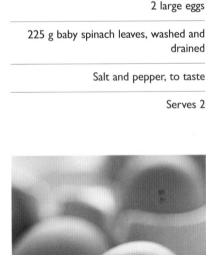

# FISH PIE WITH ROSTI TOPPING

*A crisp potato and red onion topping hides a rich creamy mixture of smoked haddock, petits pois and French beans.*

1  Cook the potatoes, whole, in their skins, in plenty of boiling salted water for 15 minutes. Drain well and set aside to cool.

2  Meanwhile, heat the oil in a saucepan and cook the onion for 5–7 minutes, until soft and lightly golden. Peel and coarsely grate the potatoes into a sieve, squeezing out any excess moisture. Mix the potatoes, onion and chopped herbs together and season well. Set aside.

3  Put the haddock, peppercorns and stock in a large pan. Bring to the boil, then cover and simmer gently for about 5–7 minutes, or until the fish is just tender. Remove the fish from the stock and flake the flesh, discarding the skin and any bones. Set aside.

4  Cook the petits pois and French beans in boiling salted water for 4–5 minutes, or until just tender. Drain well.

5  Heat the oven to 200°C, gas mark 6. In a saucepan, gently heat the mascarpone and cook for 5–7 minutes until it has thickened. Put the fish, petits pois and French beans in a shallow ovenproof dish and pour over the cheese sauce. Gently mix and season to taste.

6  Mix the potato and onion with the melted butter and spoon over the fish mixture, making sure it covers the filling. Cook in the oven for 20–25 minutes, until golden brown.

**FOR THE TOPPING**

750 g large waxy potatoes

2 tablespoons olive oil

1 large red onion, thinly sliced

1 tablespoon fresh mixed herbs, chopped

Salt and pepper, to taste

**FOR THE FILLING**

450 g smoked haddock fillet

6 whole peppercorns

200 ml fish or vegetable stock

125 g frozen petits pois

125 g French beans, halved

500 g mascarpone cheese

Salt and pepper, to taste

25 g melted butter

Serves 6

# DEEP-FRIED WHITEBAIT

*Like all fish that are eaten with their bones, whitebait are an excellent source of calcium. Mixing a little plain yogurt with the mayonnaise helps to reduce the fat content and boost the calcium content.*

1  Mix the paprika with the flour and season to taste. Toss the whitebait in the seasoned flour.

2  Heat the oil in a deep fat fryer to 190°C. Add the whitebait to the hot oil in batches, cooking each batch for about 3 minutes, until the fish is golden brown. Drain on absorbent kitchen paper and keep warm while you cook the rest.

3  Mix the mayonnaise, yogurt, chives and lemon zest together. Garnish the whitebait with lemon wedges and serve with the yogurt dip.

1 tablespoon paprika

6 tablespoons plain flour

Salt and pepper, to taste

450 g whitebait

Oil, for deep-frying

5 tablespoons mayonnaise

3 tablespoons plain yogurt

2 tablespoon fresh chives, chopped

Zest of 1 lemon

Lemon wedges, to garnish

Serves 4

# MONKFISH KEBABS WITH ROASTED VEGETABLES & PESTO

## FOR THE ROASTED VEGETABLES

2 red peppers, deseeded and cut into bite-sized pieces

I large aubergine, cut into bite-sized pieces

2 small red onions, peeled and cut into quarters

2 large courgettes, sliced into bite-sized pieces

6 cloves garlic, peeled

4 tablespoons olive oil

Salt and pepper, to taste

## FOR THE PESTO

85 g fresh watercress, chopped

I clove garlic, peeled

50 g Parmesan cheese, freshly grated

6 tablespoons olive oil

## FOR THE KEBABS

450 g monkfish, cut into 24 bite-sized pieces

6 slices Parma ham, cut into strips

16 cherry tomatoes

Serves 4

*Using watercress instead of basil in the pesto helps to boost the calcium content. Watercress is also rich in vitamin C and betacarotene, and provides useful amounts of iron.*

1 Preheat the oven to 220°C, gas mark 7. Place the peppers, aubergine, onions, courgettes and garlic in a large roasting tin, drizzle over the olive oil and mix well. Season and place in the oven for 20–30 minutes, until the vegetables are tender.

2 To make the pesto, place the watercress, garlic, Parmesan cheese and olive oil in a blender or food processor and blend until smooth.

3 Wrap each piece of monkfish in a strip of Parma ham. Thread 3 pieces onto each of 8 wood skewers, alternating with cherry tomatoes. (The skewers should be soaked in water for 30 minutes beforehand to prevent burning.)

4 Brush the kebabs with a little oil and place under a hot grill for 3–4 minutes. Turn and cook for a further 3 minutes until cooked through. Serve the kebabs with the roasted vegetables and pesto.

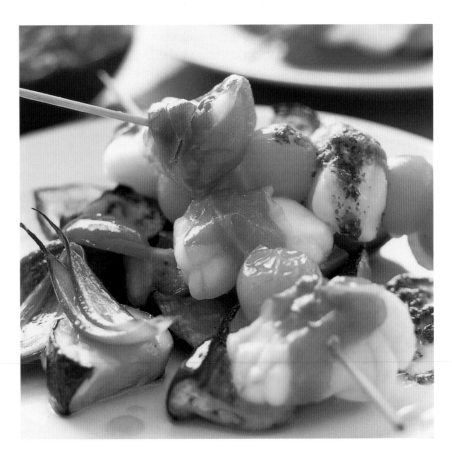

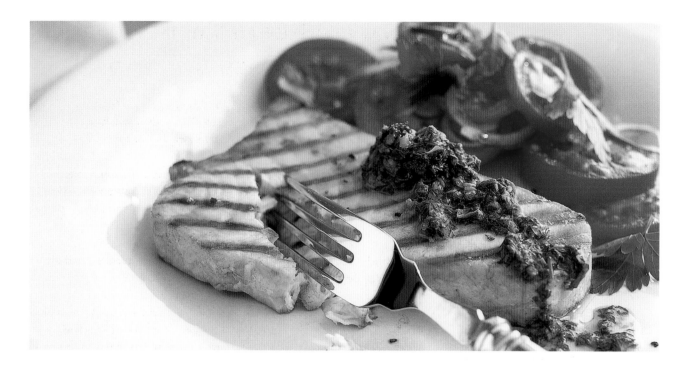

# GRIDDLED SWORDFISH WITH SALSA VERDE

*Salsa verde is a fresh, tasty sauce, which works particularly well with white fish. Serve this dish with a simple tomato salad. Anchovies are a useful source of calcium particularly for people who don't eat dairy products.*

1   To make the salsa verde, place the anchovies, capers and garlic in a food processor and blend for 30 seconds. Add the mint, basil, parsley, mustard, lemon juice and olive oil and blend until smooth.

2   Brush a griddle pan with a little olive oil and heat. When the pan is hot, add the swordfish steaks and cook for 4–5 minutes. Turn and cook for a further 4–5 minutes. Serve with the salsa verde.

4 anchovy fillets, drained and roughly chopped

1 tablespoon capers, drained and rinsed

1 clove garlic, peeled

15 g fresh mint leaves

15 g fresh basil leaves

15 g fresh flat-leaf parsley leaves or 30 g watercress

1 teaspoon Dijon mustard

Juice of 1 lemon

6 tablespoons olive oil, plus extra for brushing

4 swordfish steaks

Serves 4

# PRAWN & SPINACH ROULADE

*This attractive roulade makes a great summer meal. Make sure the spinach is drained thoroughly before adding it to the sauce.*

50 g butter, plus extra for greasing

125 g frozen chopped spinach, thawed and drained

50 g plain flour

300 ml full-fat milk

2 eggs, separated

### FOR THE FILLING

250 g mascarpone cheese

4 spring onions, finely chopped

2 sun-dried tomatoes, finely chopped

225 g peeled prawns, cooked

Salt and pepper, to taste

Serves 6

1  Grease and line a 33 × 23 cm Swiss roll tin with non-stick baking parchment. Preheat the oven to 220°C, gas mark 7.

2  Melt the butter in a saucepan and stir in the spinach and flour. Cook for 1 minute, then add the milk. Bring to the boil, stirring continuously, then simmer for 2–3 minutes. Remove from the heat and beat in the egg yolks. In a clean bowl, stiffly whisk the egg whites, then fold into the mixture.

3  Spoon the mixture into the tin and spread out evenly with a palate knife. Bake in the oven for about 15 minutes, or until well-risen and firm to the touch. Turn out on to a sheet of non-stick baking parchment and peel off the lining paper. Leave covered with a damp cloth for 20 minutes to cool.

4  Meanwhile, mix together the mascarpone cheese, spring onions, sun-dried tomatoes and prawns. Season well, then cover until the roulade is cool.

5  Spread the roulade with the prawn filling, leaving a 2.5 cm border. Starting at one long side, gently roll up the roulade, using the paper to help. Serve in thick slices with a crisp green salad.

# PENNE WITH PRAWNS & ASPARAGUS

*The lemon in this pasta enhances the flavours of the asparagus and the prawns and makes this a light, refreshing dish.*

150 g penne or other pasta

125 g asparagus tips

4 tablespoons olive oil

3 tablespoons Parmesan cheese, freshly grated

Zest and juice of 1 large lemon

2 tablespoons fresh chives, snipped

200 g peeled prawns, cooked

Serves 2

1  Cook the pasta according to the manufacturer's instructions. About 4–5 minutes before it has finished cooking, add the asparagus and continue to cook until the asparagus is tender. Drain well and return to the pan.

2  Meanwhile, whisk together the olive oil, Parmesan cheese, lemon zest and juice and chives.

3  Stir in the lemon dressing and prawns. Cook, stirring continuously, for 4–5 minutes, or until the prawns are hot.

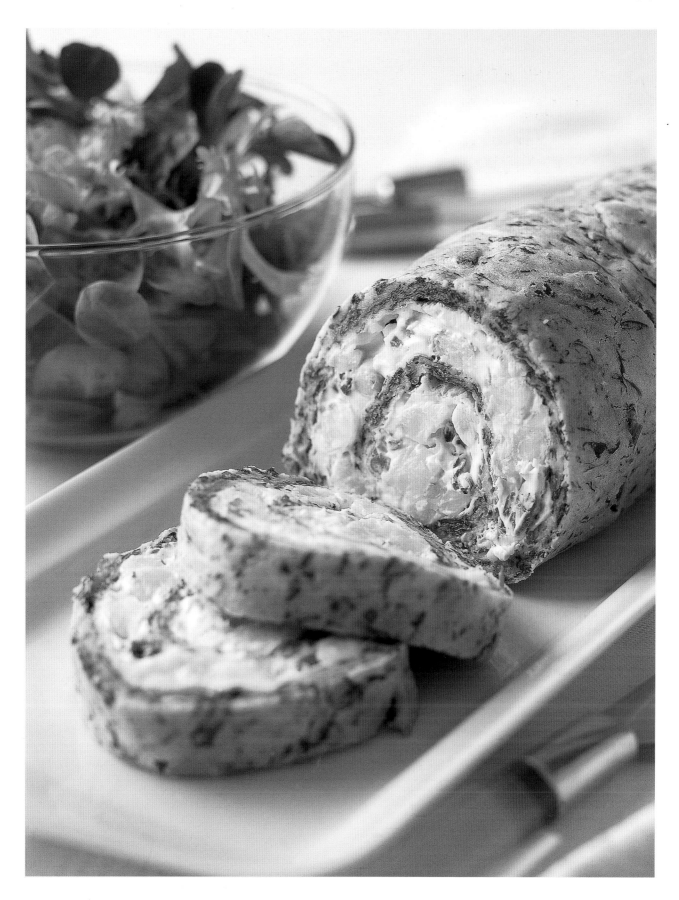

# WARM LENTIL & FETA SALAD

225 g puy lentils

1 clove garlic, peeled

1 bay leaf

4 tablespoons olive oil

2 tablespoons balsamic vinegar

1 clove garlic, crushed

½ teaspoon salt

½ teaspoon English mustard powder

300 g cherry tomatoes, sliced in half

3 tablespoons fresh parsley, chopped

200 g feta cheese, crumbled

Salt and pepper, to taste

Serves 4

*The subtle flavour of the puy lentils is perfectly complemented by the cool feta cheese, which is also a good source of calcium.*

1 Place the lentils, garlic and bay leaf in a saucepan. Cover with plenty of water and cook for 30–40 minutes, or until the lentils are just soft.

2 Whisk the olive oil, balsamic vinegar, garlic, salt and mustard powder together in a small bowl, to make a dressing.

3 Drain the lentils and transfer to a warm serving dish. Stir in the tomatoes, parsley and dressing. Add the feta cheese, season to taste and serve.

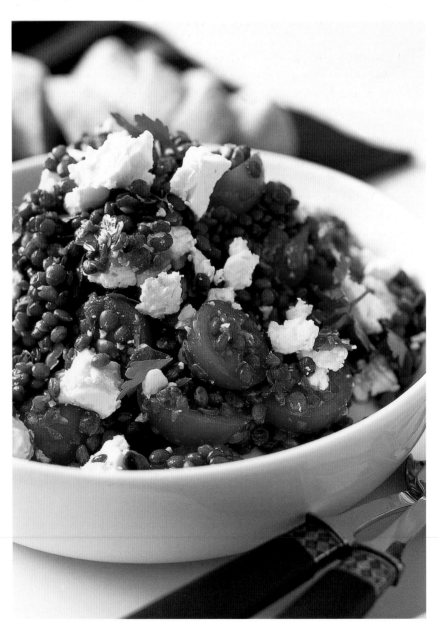

# SPICED SPINACH, LENTIL & FETA FILO PIE

*When working with filo it is essential to keep the sheets covered with a damp cloth as you work to prevent them drying out and becoming brittle.*

1　Preheat the oven to 190°C, gas mark 5. Lightly grease a 22.5 cm springform tin and set aside.

2　To make the filling, heat the oil in a saucepan. Add the onion, garlic, ground coriander and cumin and fry gently for 10 minutes. Stir in the lentils, cover and heat through for 4–5 minutes, then mash with a fork. Transfer to a bowl and leave to cool slightly.

3　Meanwhile, cook the spinach in a large saucepan for 2–3 minutes until just wilted – there is no need to add extra water as enough clings to the leaves after washing. Refresh under cold running water. Squeeze out any excess water, shred the leaves and add to the bowl with the spiced lentils.

4　Stir the eggs into the mixture, then add the feta, Parmesan cheese, fresh coriander and season to taste. Toss to mix, then set aside.

5　Lay the filo pastry in the base of the prepared tin and brush with a little of the butter. Make sure the filo forms a solid base, but leave plenty overhanging the edges of the tin. Spoon in the filling and fold over the filo to cover the topping completely.

6　Gently scrunch the remaining sheets of filo and arrange on top of the pie to give a ruffled effect. Brush with the remaining butter. Bake for 30–35 minutes until golden. Allow to cool slightly before turning out. Cut into wedges and serve.

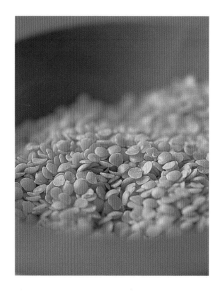

3 tablespoons olive oil, plus extra for greasing

1 medium red onion, finely chopped

3 garlic cloves, crushed

2 teaspoons ground coriander

1 teaspoon ground cumin

2 x 300 g can lentils, drained

350 g baby spinach leaves, washed

2 eggs, beaten

175 g feta cheese, crumbled

2 tablespoons Parmesan cheese, freshly grated

4 tablespoons fresh coriander, chopped

Salt and pepper, to taste

12 sheets of filo pastry (or 6 large sheets, halved)

75 g unsalted butter, melted

Serves 6

# CHEESE & LEEK SAUSAGES

175 g fine white breadcrumbs

125 g Caerphilly or Cheddar cheese

1 small leek, trimmed and finely chopped

1 tablespoon fresh parsley, finely chopped

Pinch of mustard powder

Salt and pepper, to taste

1 egg, beaten

2–3 tablespoons milk

Plain flour, for coating

Vegetable oil, for frying or brushing

Serves 4

*These are ideal for children, but adults are sure to love them, too. They provide a good alternative to meat-filled sausages.*

1  In a large bowl, mix together the breadcrumbs, cheese, leek, parsley and mustard powder. Season to taste. Add the egg and mix thoroughly, then add enough milk to bind the mixture together.

2  Divide the mixture into 8 and shape into sausages.

3  If shallow frying, roll the sausages in the flour. Heat a little oil in a large non-stick frying pan, add the sausages and fry for about 5 minutes, or until golden brown. Alternatively, lightly brush the sausages with a little oil and cook under a hot grill for about 3–4 minutes, turning occasionally. Serve hot or cold.

# VEGETABLE PATTIES

350 g potatoes, peeled and cut into even-sized pieces

3 tablespoons semi-skimmed milk

350 g mixed vegetables

3 tablespoons vegetable oil

1 small onion, finely chopped

1 clove garlic, crushed

200 g Cheddar cheese, grated

Salt and pepper, to taste

25 g plain flour, for dusting

1 egg, beaten

125 g fine white breadcrumbs

Serves 4

*You can use any mixed vegetables you like in these patties, such as carrots, broccoli, spinach, peas and sweetcorn. They are delicious served with a tomato salad.*

1  Cook the potatoes in boiling, salted water for 15–20 minutes. Drain well, then mash with the milk. Steam the mixed vegetables and chop finely.

2  Heat 1 tablespoon of the oil in a large non-stick frying pan. Add the onion and garlic and cook over a medium heat for 5 minutes until soft.

3  Stir the cooked vegetables, onion and garlic mixture and the grated cheese into the mashed potato. Season to taste, cover and chill for 1 hour.

4  Turn the mixture onto a floured surface and shape into 8 rounds. Dip the patties into the beaten egg and coat in the breadcrumbs. Chill for 15 minutes.

5  Heat the remaining oil and fry the patties, in batches, over a medium heat for 3–4 minutes on each side, or until golden brown.

BUBBLE & SQUEAK

The vegetable mixture also makes a delicious bubble and squeak. Follow the recipe up until the end of step 3. Heat 1 tablespoon of oil in a large non-stick frying pan, add the mixture and fry until heated through and browned.

# SPICED TOFU BURGERS

*Using tofu for these vegetarian burgers ensures that they are lower in fat than those that contain a large quantity of nuts. Serve in a burger bun with mayonnaise, lettuce and slices of tomato, not forgetting the oven chips.*

1 Heat the oil in a large non-stick frying pan. Add the carrots and onion and cook, stirring continuously, for 3–4 minutes, or until the vegetables are soft. Add the ground coriander, garlic, curry paste and tomato purée. Increase the heat and cook for 2 minutes, stirring all the time.

2 Mash the tofu with a potato masher, then stir into the vegetables along with the breadcrumbs and nuts. Season well and stir until the mixture starts to stick together.

3 With floured hands, shape the mixture into 4 burgers. Heat a little of the oil in a large non-stick frying pan and fry the burgers for 3–4 minutes on each side, or until golden brown. Alternatively, to grill the burgers, brush them with a little oil and cook under a preheated grill for about 3 minutes on each side. Drain on kitchen paper and serve.

1 tablespoon vegetable oil

1 large carrot, grated

1 large red onion, grated

2 teaspoons ground coriander

1 garlic clove, peeled and crushed

1 teaspoon hot curry paste

1 teaspoon sun-dried tomato purée

225 g tofu, drained

25 g wholemeal breadcrumbs

25 g mixed nuts, toasted and finely chopped

Salt and pepper, to taste

Plain flour, for dusting

Vegetable oil, for frying or grilling

Makes 4 burgers

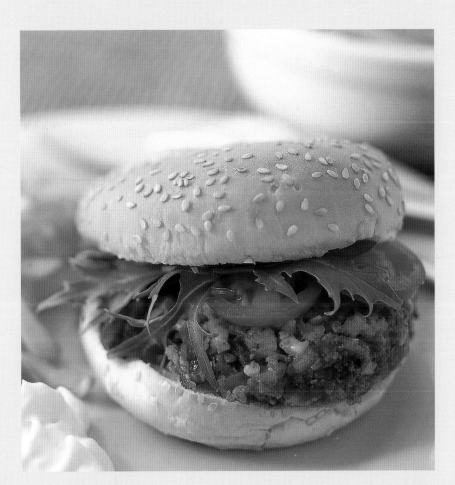

# ROASTED THAI-STYLE TOFU WITH STIR-FRIED VEGETABLES

450 g tofu, drained

1 garlic clove, peeled and finely chopped

2 tablespoons hoisin sauce

2 tablespoons dark soy sauce

1 tablespoon sherry vinegar

1 tablespoon sweet chilli sauce

1 tablespoon runny honey

1 teaspoon sesame oil

### FOR THE STIR-FRY

3 tablespoons sunflower oil

1 teaspoon sesame oil

1 medium red onion, roughly chopped

2 carrots, cut into matchsticks

1 red pepper, thinly sliced

175 g broccoli florets

125 g chestnut mushrooms, quartered

6 spring onions, sliced

125 g sugar snap peas

Toasted sesame seeds, to garnish

Serves 4

*Tofu is ideal for the modern healthy diet because it is low in fat and is a good source of protein. Here, the tofu is glazed in a Thai-style sauce and served with a selection of stir-fried vegetables. Egg noodles or plain boiled rice make ideal accompaniments.*

1 Preheat the oven to 220°C, gas mark 8. Cut the tofu into 2.5 cm cubes and place in a shallow roasting tin. Mix together the garlic, hoisin sauce, soy sauce, sherry vinegar, chilli sauce, honey and sesame oil. Pour two-thirds of the marinade over the tofu and toss well, making sure the tofu is coated thoroughly. Roast for 25 minutes, turning once, until the tofu is deep golden brown and glazed.

2 Meanwhile, heat both oils in a wok or large non-stick frying pan. Add the red onion, carrots, red pepper, broccoli and mushrooms and stir-fry for 3 minutes. Add the spring onions and sugar snap peas and stir-fry for a further 2 minutes.

3 Add 2 tablespoons of water to the remaining glaze and add this to the stir-fried vegetables. Cook for another 2–3 minutes until the vegetables are just tender, then stir in the roasted tofu. Garnish with toasted sesame seeds and serve immediately.

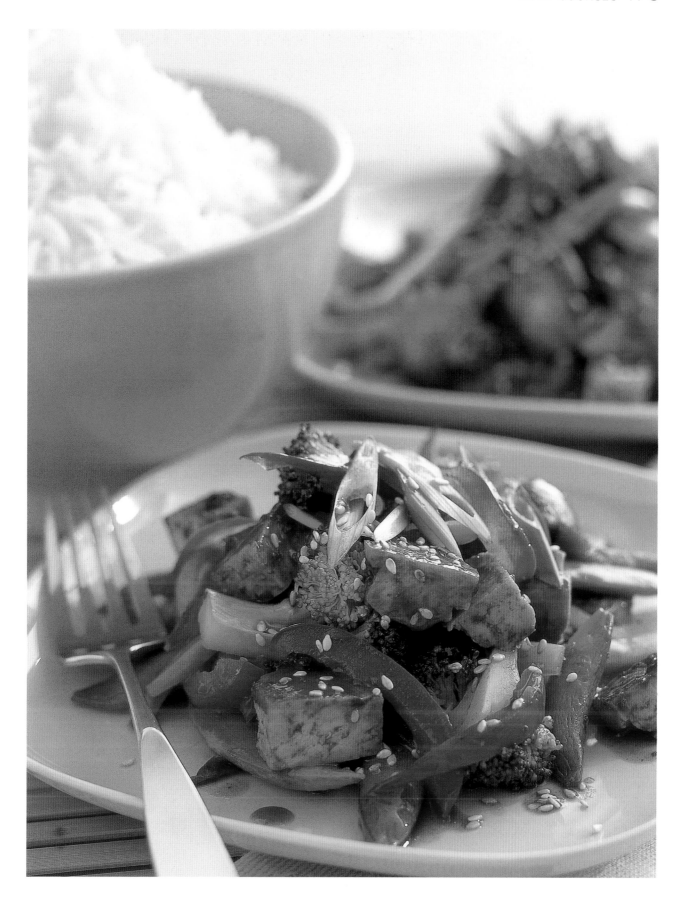

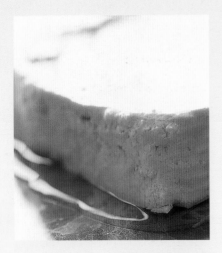

# MARINATED TOFU WITH SATAY SAUCE

*Pressed tofu is ideal for marinating because it contains less liquid and will, therefore, absorb more flavour. The satay sauce can be made in advance and reheated before serving.*

1   Cut the tofu into 1 cm pieces. In a shallow dish, mix together the onion, soy sauce and sugar. Add the tofu pieces and toss, ensuring that the tofu is thoroughly coated. Cover and leave to marinate for at least 1 hour. Soak 8 wooden skewers in cold water for 30 minutes.

2   Meanwhile, for the satay sauce, heat the oil in a saucepan and add the garlic and chilli powder. Cook, stirring, for 1–2 minutes. Add the peanut butter, sugar and lemon zest, along with 300 ml water. Bring to a simmer and cook for 4–5 minutes until the sauce thickens.

3   Heat the grill to high. Thread the tofu onto 8 skewers. Cook for 3–4 minutes on each side, turning occasionally until browned.

4   Serve on a bed of salad leaves, onions and carrot chunks, accompanied by the satay sauce.

---

**GRILLED VEGETABLES WITH SATAY SAUCE**
Grill a selection of vegetables, such as peppers, tomatoes, courgettes, onions or shallots and serve with the satay sauce.

250 g pressed tofu

1 small onion, finely chopped

3 tablespoons dark soy sauce

1 teaspoon dark muscovado sugar

### FOR THE SATAY SAUCE

1 tablespoon vegetable oil

1 clove garlic, peeled and crushed

2 teaspoons chilli powder

225 g crunchy peanut butter

1 tablespoon dark muscovado sugar

Zest of 1 large lemon

### TO SERVE

Selection of salad leaves, chopped onion and carrot chunks

Serves 4

# HOT SPICED CHICKPEAS

*This dish is delicious warm, accompanied by crusty wholemeal bread,
but can also be served cold with a wild rocket leaf salad.*

1   Heat the oil in a large saucepan and sauté the onions for 5–7 minutes,
    until soft.

2   Add the turmeric and cumin seeds and fry for 1 minute, stirring
    frequently. Add the chickpeas, tomatoes, lemon juice and coriander and
    sauté for 4–5 minutes until heated through.

3   Season well and serve garnished with coriander leaves and a sprinkling
    of cayenne pepper.

1 tablespoon vegetable oil

1 large red onion, roughly chopped

2 teaspoons ground turmeric

1 tablespoon cumin seeds

2 x 400 g cans chickpeas, drained
and rinsed

450 g cherry tomatoes, halved

1 tablespoon lemon juice

4 tablespoons fresh coriander, chopped

Salt and pepper, to taste

Fresh coriander leaves, to garnish

Cayenne pepper, to garnish

Serves 6

# CHICKPEA & POTATO STEW

*A quick and easy stew using canned chickpeas and potatoes
flavoured with Indian spices. Serve with boiled pilau rice.*

1   In a large saucepan, heat the oil and cook the onion for 5 minutes until soft.

2   Add the garlic and curry paste and cook for 30 seconds, stirring frequently.
    Stir in the potato, chickpeas and chilli and season well. Add the stock and
    150 ml water. Simmer for 30 minutes.

3   Add the spring onions, 3 tablespoons of chopped coriander, lime juice and
    garam masala. Reheat and simmer for 2–3 minutes. Season to taste.
    Garnish with the remaining chopped coriander and serve.

CHICKPEA AND SWEET POTATO STEW
For an interesting variation on this recipe, replace the potato with sweet potato
which will give it a more mellow flavour.

2 tablespoons sunflower oil

2 medium red onions, chopped

4 cloves garlic, peeled and chopped

2 tablespoons medium-hot curry paste

450 g potatoes, diced

2 x 400 g cans chickpeas, drained
and rinsed

1 red chilli, deseeded and chopped

Salt and pepper, to taste

300 ml vegetable stock

6 spring onions, chopped

4 tablespoons fresh coriander, chopped

Juice of 1 lime

1 teaspoon garam masala

Serves 4

# MIXED BEANS WITH A CORNMEAL TOPPING

FOR THE BEANS

1 tablespoon olive oil

1 small onion, finely chopped

2 garlic cloves, peeled and finely chopped

400 g can chopped tomatoes

200 ml vegetable stock

2 tablespoons dark soy sauce

3 tablespoons dark brown sugar

1 tablespoon mild mustard

2 x 400 g cans of mixed beans, rinsed and drained

FOR THE TOPPING

50 g self-raising flour

50 g cornmeal (polenta)

¼ teaspoon salt

½ teaspoon baking powder

5 tablespoons full-fat milk

2 eggs, separated

1 tablespoon olive oil

125 g Cheddar cheese, grated

Serves 4

*Canned beans and pulses are a good store cupboard ingredient. They are rich in soluble fibre (the type that helps reduce cholesterol levels) and are also a useful source of calcium.*

1 Heat 1 tablespoon of the oil in a saucepan. Add the onion and garlic and cook for 5 minutes until soft. Add the tomatoes, stock and soy sauce. Bring to the boil, then reduce to a fast simmer and cook for about 15 minutes, or until the sauce begins to thicken.

2 Add the sugar, mustard and mixed beans. Continue to cook for a further 5 minutes, until the beans are hot.

3 Preheat the oven to 200°C, gas mark 6. Meanwhile, make the topping; mix the flour, cornmeal, salt, baking powder, milk, egg yolks, oil and 75 g of the cheese in a bowl. Beat together to make a fairly stiff batter, adding a little extra milk if necessary.

4 Whisk the egg whites in a clean bowl until stiff, then, using a metal spoon, fold carefully into the batter.

5 Transfer the beans to a shallow ovenproof dish and spoon over the topping. Sprinkle over the remaining Cheddar cheese and cook for 20 minutes, until the topping is golden brown and well risen.

# BUTTERNUT SQUASH & GRUYERE RISOTTO

*You can use any type of squash or pumpkin to make this delicious creamy risotto. The secret of a good risotto is to keep it simmering slowly while you add the stock a little at a time, so it cooks evenly. Arborio rice is the best-known Italian rice and is ideal for risotto – its plump, long grains absorb liquid without losing their bite.*

1 Heat the oil in a large saucepan, add the leeks, garlic, chilli, rosemary and sage and cook for 5 minutes until soft.

2 Add the rice and stir-fry for 1 minute until all the grains are glossy. Bring the vegetable stock to a steady simmer in another saucepan.

3 Add the butternut squash and stir well. Pour in 150 ml of the hot stock and stir over a medium heat until absorbed. Gradually add the remaining stock, a ladleful at a time, stirring occasionally, making sure each addition is absorbed before adding the next. Continue until the rice is tender and all the stock absorbed – this should take about 25 minutes.

4 Remove from the heat and stir in 100 g of the Gruyère cheese and the cream. Cover and allow to stand for 5 minutes. Season well to taste.

5 Top with the remaining 25 g of the Gruyère cheese and a grinding of black pepper. Garnish with small fresh rosemary sprigs and Gruyère shavings.

4 tablespoons extra virgin olive oil

2 leeks, trimmed and thinly sliced

2 garlic cloves, finely chopped

1 red chilli, deseeded and thinly sliced

1 tablespoon fresh rosemary, chopped

1 tablespoon fresh sage, chopped

225 g arborio rice

1 litre vegetable stock

450 g butternut squash, peeled, deseeded and chopped

125 g Gruyère cheese, grated

4 tablespoons double cream

Salt and pepper, to taste

Small fresh rosemary sprigs, to garnish

Gruyère shavings, to garnish

Serves 4

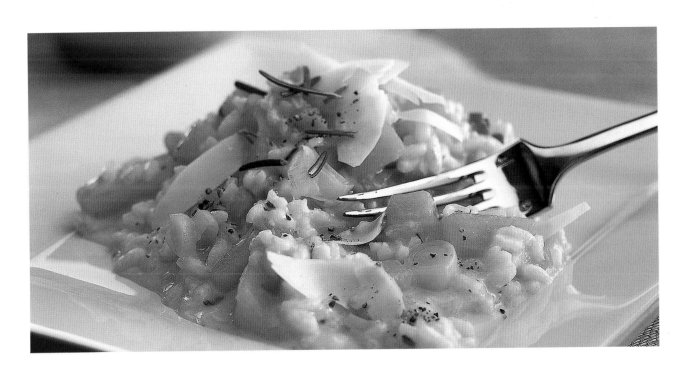

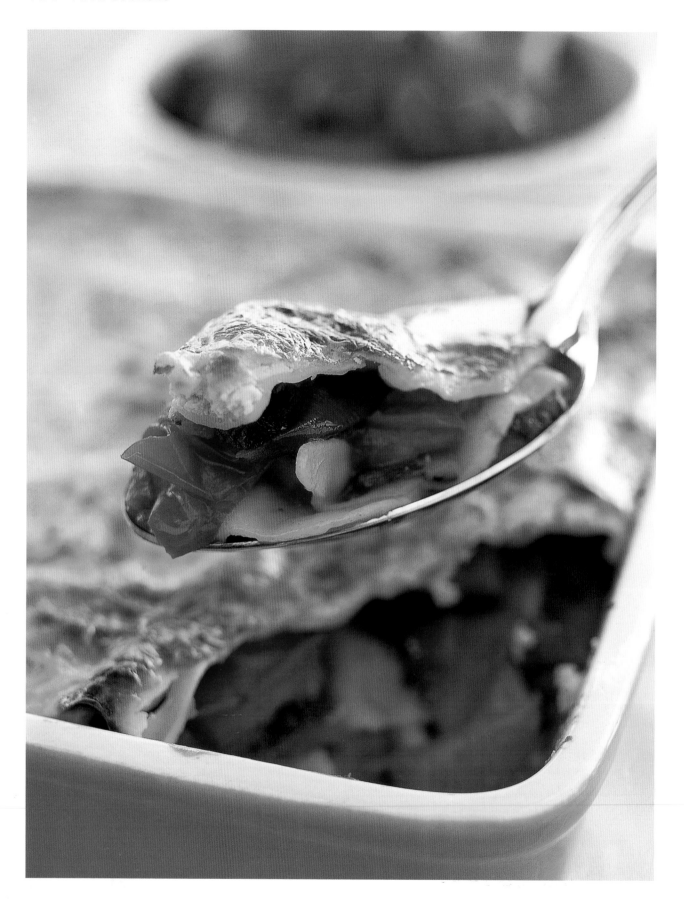

# ROASTED VEGETABLE LASAGNE

*Served with a tomato and basil salad, this recipe provides a healthy, balanced meal. You can use pre-cooked lasagne sheets, but add a little extra liquid to the vegetable and tomato mixture.*

| 1 | Preheat the oven to 190°C, gas mark 5. Place the chopped vegetables in a large shallow roasting tin. Toss in the oil and season well. Roast for 25–30 minutes until slightly blackened. Leave to cool slightly. |

2   Meanwhile, mix together the ricotta cheese with the egg, milk and 4 tablespoons of the Parmesan cheese. Season well and set aside.

3   Spoon the roasted vegetables into a large bowl and mix with the canned tomatoes (use those with added garlic and herbs for extra flavour) and basil. Spoon a layer of vegetable and tomato mixture over the base of a lightly greased ovenproof dish and cover with a layer of lasagne sheets.

4   Continue with another layer of the vegetable and tomato mixture, then another layer of lasagne. Repeat this process once more, then spread the ricotta cheese mixture evenly over the top and sprinkle with the remaining Parmesan cheese. Bake for 30 minutes or until golden brown and bubbling.

5   Leave the lasagne to stand for 5 minutes before serving.

1 large courgette, roughly chopped

1 red pepper, deseeded and chopped

1 red onion, roughly chopped

1 small aubergine, chopped

2 tablespoons olive oil

Salt and pepper, to taste

250 g ricotta cheese

1 egg

4 tablespoons full-fat milk

6 tablespoons Parmesan cheese, grated

2 x 400 g cans chopped tomatoes

2 tablespoons fresh basil, chopped

8–10 sheets fresh lasagne

Serves 4

# PAPPARDELLE WITH SPICY TOMATO SAUCE & RICOTTA

*Ricotta cheese is surprisingly low in fat compared with many other cheeses, but still provides useful amounts of calcium. The creaminess of the ricotta perfectly balances the heat of the sauce. If time is short, use ready-made arrabbiata sauce instead of making your own tomato sauce.*

1   Heat the oil in large saucepan, add the onion, garlic, ground coriander and cumin and cook for 5 minutes, or until the onions are soft. Add the tomatoes, tomato purée, red wine and seasoning, bring to the boil, then simmer for about 30 minutes, or until the sauce has reduced by about half.

2   Cook the pasta according to the packet instructions and drain well.

3   Transfer the pasta to a serving dish, spoon over the tomato sauce, then stir in the ricotta cheese. Garnish with fresh basil and serve immediately.

1 tablespoon olive oil

1 large red onion, finely chopped

1 clove garlic, peeled and finely chopped

1 teaspoon ground coriander

1 teaspoon ground cumin

2 x 400 g cans chopped tomatoes

1 tablespoon tomato purée

150 ml red wine

Salt and pepper, to taste

250 g pappardelle, or other pasta

200 g ricotta cheese

Fresh basil, chopped, to garnish

Serves 4

# BROCCOLI & GRUYERE SOUFFLE

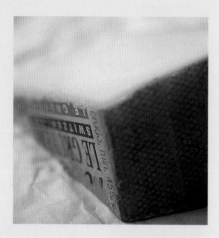

*Broccoli is good source of vitamin K, which is an important nutrient for bone health. It also provides useful amounts of calcium, so is particularly good for people on a dairy-free diet.*

1 Preheat the oven to 180°C, gas mark 4. Grease 6 ramekin dishes and place on a baking tray. Steam the broccoli over a pan of boiling water for 8 minutes until tender.

2 Melt the butter in a saucepan, stir in the flour and cook for 1 minute. Gradually stir in the milk and bring to the boil. Cook, stirring continuously, until the mixture has thickened.

3 Pour the sauce into a food processor, add the broccoli and purée until the mixture is smooth.

4 Transfer the mixture to a bowl, allow to cool slightly, then stir in the egg yolks and Gruyère cheese. Season to taste.

5 In a clean bowl, whisk the egg whites until stiff, then lightly fold into the sauce mixture.

6 Spoon into the ramekin dishes, transfer to the oven and cook for 20–25 minutes, or until the soufflés are just firm to the touch. Serve immediately.

Butter, for greasing

225 g broccoli florets

40 g butter

3 tablespoons plain flour

200 ml full-fat milk

3 eggs, separated

125 g Gruyère cheese, grated

Salt and pepper, to taste

Serves 6

## SPINACH AND GRUYERE SOUFFLE

Replace the broccoli with 225 g cooked spinach. Squeeze any excess moisture from the spinach and follow the instructions above.

# MEDITERRANEAN STUFFED PEPPERS WITH COUSCOUS

*Couscous is an ideal accompaniment to these tasty and healthy stuffed peppers. They can also be served on top of toasted ciabatta rubbed with garlic, accompanied by a rocket salad.*

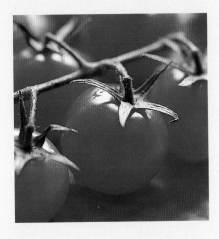

1. Preheat the oven to 180°C, gas mark 4. Cut the peppers in half through the stalks. Scoop out the seeds and the white ribs, leaving the stalk intact. Put the pepper halves cut-side up into a large roasting tin and set aside.

2. To remove the tomato skins, mark a cross in the top of each one and put them into a bowl. Cover with boiling water and leave for 1 minute, then drain. Leave to cool slightly then peel off the skin and cut the tomatoes into wedges.

3. Mix the tomato wedges, garlic, capers, olives and oregano together, then spoon into the pepper halves. Drizzle over the olive oil and season well.

4. Roast for 35 minutes. Remove from the oven and scatter over the feta and pine nuts or shredded almonds. Return to the oven and cook for a further 10 minutes, or until the feta has melted and the nuts are lightly golden.

5. Meanwhile, put the couscous into a large bowl and pour over the boiling water or vegetable stock. Leave for about 5 minutes until the stock is absorbed and the couscous soft. Fluff up the couscous mixture with a fork and toss in the chopped parsley, spring onions, lemon zest and a drizzle of olive oil.

6. To serve, place a little couscous and 2 roasted pepper halves onto each of 4 serving plates. Garnish with parsley and a grinding of black pepper.

## FOR THE STUFFED PEPPERS

4 large red peppers

12 cherry tomatoes, halved

3 cloves garlic, peeled and thinly sliced

1 teaspoon capers, drained and rinsed

8 pitted black olives, roughly chopped

1 tablespoon fresh oregano, chopped

4 tablespoons virgin olive oil

Salt and pepper, to taste

125 g feta cheese, crumbled

2 tablespoons pine nuts or shredded almonds

## FOR THE COUSCOUS

225 g couscous

300 ml boiling water or hot vegetable stock

2 tablespoons fresh flat-leaf parsley, chopped, plus extra to garnish

4 spring onions, shredded

Zest of 1 lemon

Olive oil, for drizzling

Serves 4

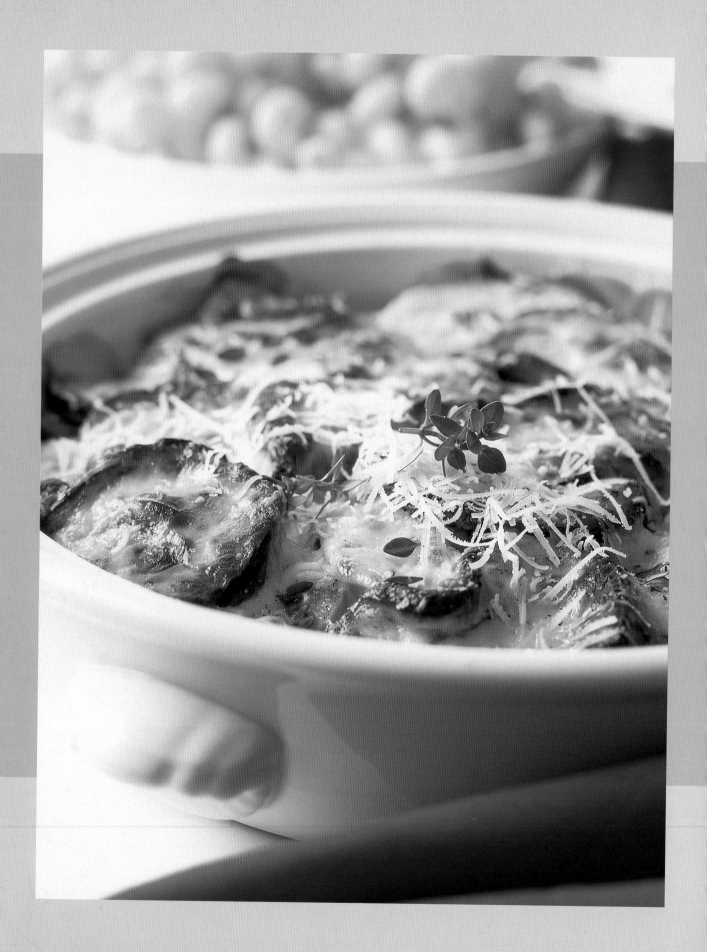

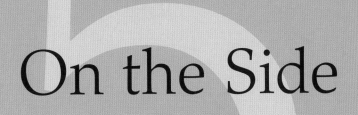

# 5 On the Side

ACCOMPANIMENTS CAN SOMETIMES
BECOME A SECOND THOUGHT WHEN
PREPARING A MEAL, SO THIS CHAPTER
OFFERS CREATIVE IDEAS FOR
VEGETABLE SIDE DISHES AND SALADS
THAT WILL BOOST THE FLAVOUR AND
NUTRITIONAL VALUE OF ANY DISH.

# FRENCH BEANS WITH FETA & SUN-DRIED TOMATOES

250 g green beans, trimmed

75 g feta cheese, crumbled

50 g sun-dried tomatoes in oil, sliced into thin strips

Salt and pepper, to taste

Serves 4

*The combination of feta and sun-dried tomatoes gives this accompaniment a classic Mediterranean flavour. It works well with plain grilled meat or fish.*

1  Cook the beans in a large pan of boiling salted water for 3–4 minutes or until just tender. Drain well.

2  Toss the beans with the feta cheese and sun-dried tomatoes. Season to taste and serve.

# ROASTED BABY CARROTS WITH PARMESAN & CORIANDER TOPPING

600 g baby carrots

1 tablespoon sunflower oil

1 tablespoon unsalted butter

Salt and pepper, to taste

3 tablespoons fresh coriander, chopped

50 g Parmesan cheese, freshly grated

Serves 4

*The Parmesan cheese and coriander topping is quick and tasty and works well with most vegetables. Adding a cheesy crust is also a great way to persuade kids to eat vegetables.*

1  Preheat the oven to 200°C, gas mark 6. Put the carrots in a large saucepan of boiling water and boil for 3 minutes. Drain well.

2  Place the carrots in a shallow ovenproof dish with the oil, butter and seasoning. Roast in the oven for 15 minutes.

3  Meanwhile, mix the coriander and Parmesan cheese together in a small bowl. Remove the carrots from the oven and sprinkle with the mixture. Return to the oven for another 10 minutes, until the carrots are tender and lightly golden.

### SPICY ROAST BABY CARROTS WITH FETA

Follow steps 1 and 2 as above. With a pestle and mortar, grind together 1 teaspoon coriander seeds, 1 teaspoon ground cardamom, 1 bay leaf, 1 teaspoon cumin seeds, 6 peppercorns, 1 teaspoon hot paprika and half a cinnamon stick. Sprinkle this mixture over the roasted carrots and toss lightly, then crumble over 200 g feta cheese. Return the carrots to the oven for 10 minutes until they are tender and the cheese has melted.

# ASIAN-STYLE BROCCOLI

*Lightly steamed broccoli is a useful source of calcium. It also provides good amounts of betacarotene, vitamin C, vitamin $B_6$, folate and niacin.*

1   Cook the broccoli in a large pan of boiling salted water for 1–2 minutes. Immediately plunge the broccoli into ice-cold water to stop it cooking further. Drain well and blot dry with absorbent kitchen paper.

2   Heat the sesame and sunflower oils in a wok or large frying pan. Add the garlic, chilli and ginger and stir-fry for 2–3 minutes. Add the broccoli and soy sauce and continue to cook for 1 minute. Sprinkle with the sesame seeds and serve.

450 g broccoli, divided into small florets

2 teaspoons sesame oil

2 teaspoons sunflower oil

1 clove garlic, peeled and finely chopped

1 red chilli, deseeded and finely chopped

1 cm fresh ginger, chopped

1 tablespoon light soy sauce

1 teaspoon sesame seeds

Serves 4

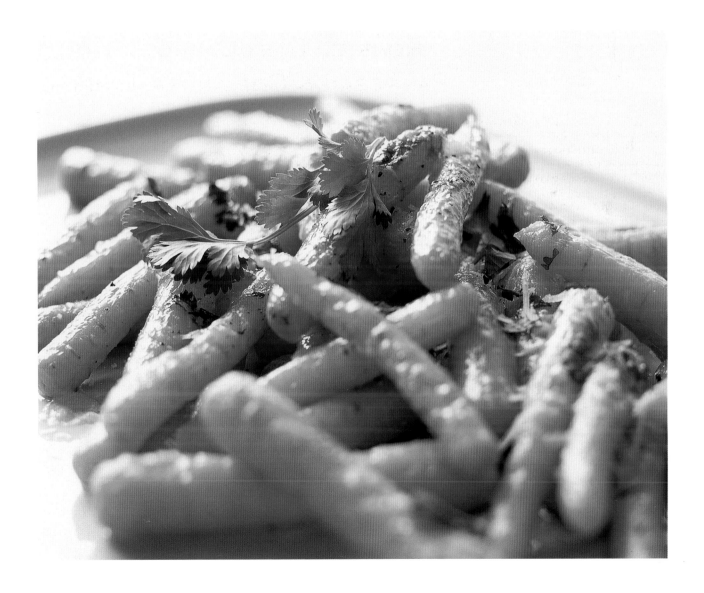

# HONEYED PARSNIPS WITH SESAME SEEDS

700 g parsnips, peeled

50 g butter

2 tablespoons honey

2 tablespoons sesame seeds, toasted

Salt and pepper, to taste

Fresh thyme sprigs, to garnish

Serves 4

*Sesame seeds are a good source of calcium, particularly for anyone following a dairy-free diet. One tablespoon of sesame seeds will provide around 10 per cent of the daily calcium requirement for women aged between 19 and 50. It also provides around 10 per cent of the daily iron requirement and 17 per cent of the daily vitamin $B_6$ requirement.*

1 Cut the parsnips in half lengthways and in half again. (If using older, tougher parsnips, cut into quarters and remove the woody cores.) Add the parsnips to a pan of boiling salted water and cook for 5 minutes.

2 Meanwhile, melt the butter in a large saucepan. Add the honey and heat gently, stirring until it is dissolved.

3 Drain the parsnips, then add the honey mixture to the pan and toss well to coat the parsnips. Cook over a moderate heat for about 10 minutes, shaking the pan frequently, until the parsnips are golden brown. Sprinkle over the sesame seeds and toss through. Season to taste.

4 Transfer to a warmed serving dish and garnish with thyme sprigs.

PARSNIPS WITH A SWEET LIME GLAZE

Prepare the parsnips as in step 1. Remove the zest from 1 lime and reserve. Put the juice of the lime, 50 g butter and 25 g soft light brown sugar in a large pan and heat until the butter is melted and the sugar dissolved. Follow the recipe as above, using the sweet lime butter in place of the honey mixture. At the end of cooking, stir through 75 g walnuts instead of the sesame seeds. Garnish with the lime zest and fresh thyme sprigs. This sweet lime glaze can be used with any sweet root vegetables, such as sweet potatoes or carrots.

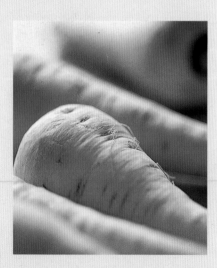

# FANTAIL ROAST POTATOES WITH SESAME SEEDS

*A roast dinner wouldn't be the same without roast potatoes, and these look attractive as well as tasting great. The sesame seeds give them a crunchy, slightly nutty taste and boost the calcium content of the dish. They are also an ideal source of potassium, which is an important ingredient for healthy bones.*

1  Preheat the oven to 180°C, gas mark 4. Place the potatoes in a large saucepan, cover with salted cold water and bring to the boil, then cook for 3 minutes. Drain well and rinse under cold running water to cool slightly.

2  Using a sharp knife, slice into each potato at 3–5 mm intervals, cutting ¾ of the way through.

3  Heat a thin layer of oil in a large roasting tin in the oven. Add the potatoes and turn over in the oil to coat. Place cut-side up and sprinkle with the sesame seeds.

4  Roast the potatoes for about 1–1¼ hours, basting occasionally. Increase the oven temperature to 220°C, gas mark 7 and roast for a further 15 minutes, until the outside of the potatoes is crisp and golden brown. Serve garnished with parsley sprigs.

1.8 kg potatoes, peeled and cut into large even-sized pieces

Salt and pepper, to taste

Vegetable oil, for basting

2 tablespoons sesame seeds

Fresh parsley sprigs, to garnish

Serves 6

## RED PESTO FANTAIL ROAST POTATOES

Follow the main recipe as above, omitting the sesame seeds. After the potatoes have been roasting for 1–1¼ hours, remove from the oven. Carefully pull the potatoes apart and spread a little red pesto between each slice – use about 3 tablespoons of pesto altogether. Close the potatoes back up and baste the tops with a little oil from the roasting tin. Increase the oven temperature, as in the main recipe, and roast for a further 15 minutes. Serve with a salad of rocket leaves, crumbled feta, cherry tomatoes, marinated red pepper and a drizzle of olive oil.

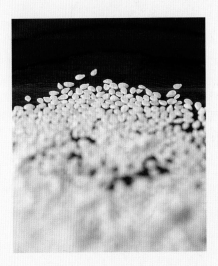

# SWEET POTATO & ANCHOVY GRATIN

450 ml full-fat milk

150 ml double cream

Butter, for greasing

1 kg sweet potatoes, sliced

2 red onions, sliced

50 g canned anchovies, drained and cut in half lengthways

2 cloves garlic, peeled and finely chopped

Salt and pepper, to taste

125 g Gruyère cheese, grated

Serves 6

*Sweet potatoes are an excellent source of betacarotene and provide good amounts of vitamin C and potassium, which are important for bone health. This dish is a perfect accompaniment for roast lamb.*

1   Put the milk and cream into a saucepan. Bring slowly to the boil, remove from the heat and set aside.

2   Preheat the oven to 200°C, gas mark 6. Grease a 1.8 litre ovenproof dish.

3   Layer the potatoes and onions in the dish with the anchovies, garlic and seasoning between the layers.

4   Pour the warm milk and cream over the potato and onion mixture. Cover the dish with foil, place on a baking sheet and bake for 1 hour. Remove the foil and scatter over the Gruyère cheese. Bake for a further 15–20 minutes until tender and golden. Serve hot.

# AUBERGINE & TOMATO GRATIN

250 g mascarpone cheese

4 tablespoons Parmesan cheese, freshly grated

Salt and pepper, to taste

2 medium aubergines

Light olive oil or vegetable oil, for frying

6 plum tomatoes, sliced

2 cloves garlic, peeled and roughly chopped

2 eggs, beaten

Fresh thyme leaves, to garnish

Serves 6

*This creamy vegetable gratin is an excellent accompaniment to lamb. It also makes a tasty vegetarian main course when served with pasta.*

1   Preheat the oven to 200°C, gas mark 6. In a saucepan, heat the mascarpone cheese for 1–2 minutes until smooth. Stir in half the Parmesan cheese and season well. Set aside.

2   Thinly slice the aubergines. Pour enough oil into a large non-stick frying pan to cover the base. Heat until the oil is very hot, then add a layer of aubergine slices – you will need to cook the aubergine in 2 batches. Fry over a moderate heat until golden brown on both sides, turning once. Remove with a slotted spoon and drain on absorbent kitchen paper. Repeat again with the remaining aubergine slices, adding more oil, if necessary.

3   Arrange alternate layers of aubergine and tomato in a greased ovenproof dish. Sprinkle a little garlic, a little salt and plenty of pepper in between each layer.

4   Beat the eggs into the cheese sauce, then slowly pour over the aubergine and tomato. Sprinkle the remaining cheese over the top. Bake for 20 minutes, or until the topping is golden and bubbling. Garnish with thyme leaves and serve hot.

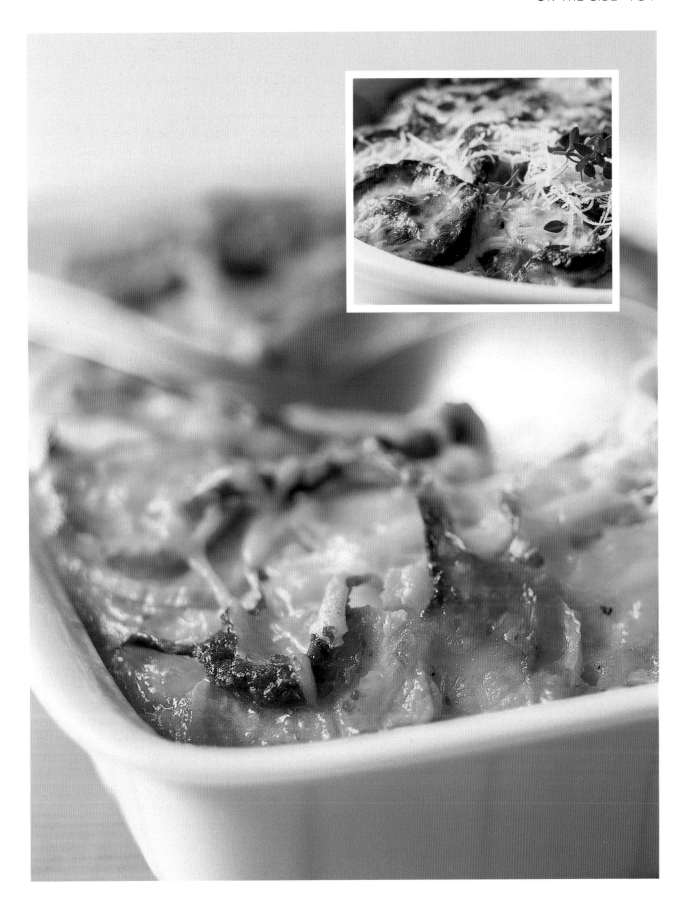

# CAULIFLOWER & BROCCOLI CHEESE

*Adding a rich, creamy mascarpone sauce to a combination of vegetables transforms this family favourite.*

350 g cauliflower florets

350 g broccoli florets

1 teaspoon vegetable oil

4 spring onions, finely shredded

500 g mascarpone cheese

125 g Cheddar cheese, grated

Salt and pepper, to taste

3 tablespoons fresh wholemeal breadcrumbs

Fresh flat-leaf parsley, roughly chopped, to garnish

Serves 6

1  Preheat the oven to 200°C, gas mark 6. Put the cauliflower and broccoli in a pan of boiling salted water. Bring back to the boil and cook for 6–7 minutes until just tender, then drain thoroughly. Place in an ovenproof dish.

2  Heat the oil in a frying pan and stir-fry the spring onions for 2–3 minutes, until softened. Add the mascarpone cheese and cook for 1–2 minutes until smooth. Stir in the half the Cheddar cheese and season well.

3  Pour the cheese sauce evenly over the cauliflower and broccoli. Sprinkle with the breadcrumbs and the remaining cheese and bake for 25 minutes, until the topping is golden and bubbling. Garnish with flat-leaf parsley and a grinding of fresh black pepper.

# APPLE, WALNUT & WATERCRESS SALAD

*Apples and walnuts are a classic combination and help to give this salad a wonderful crunchy texture. Watercress provides a useful source of calcium, particularly for people on dairy-free diets.*

50 g walnut halves

2 teaspoons sherry vinegar

3 tablespoons olive oil

1 tablespoon walnut oil

Salt and pepper, to taste

1 small red onion, peeled and thinly sliced

2 crisp green eating apples, quartered, cored and sliced

100 g watercress

Serves 4

1  To make the salad dressing, chop half the walnuts very finely by hand, or in a food processor. Place in a bowl and whisk in the vinegar, olive oil and walnut oil and season with salt and pepper. Set aside until ready to use.

2  Toss the onion, apple and watercress together in a bowl. Whisk the salad dressing and drizzle it over the salad. Sprinkle with the remaining walnut halves to serve.

# POTATO SALAD WITH BLUE CHEESE DRESSING

*A high-calcium version of a popular side dish, this is perfect as an accompaniment, and also great for a picnic or buffet lunch.*

1 Place the potatoes in a pan of boiling salted water and boil for 15–20 minutes, until cooked through.

2 Whisk together the fromage frais and milk, then stir in the cheese.

3 Drain the potatoes well and place in a serving dish. Cover with the blue cheese dressing and sprinkle with chives. Stir well to ensure the potatoes are coated with the dressing, then serve.

550 g new potatoes, sliced in half

5 tablespoons natural fromage frais

3 tablespoons semi-skimmed milk

125 g Stilton or other blue cheese, crumbled or chopped into small pieces

2 tablespoons fresh chives, chopped

Serves 4

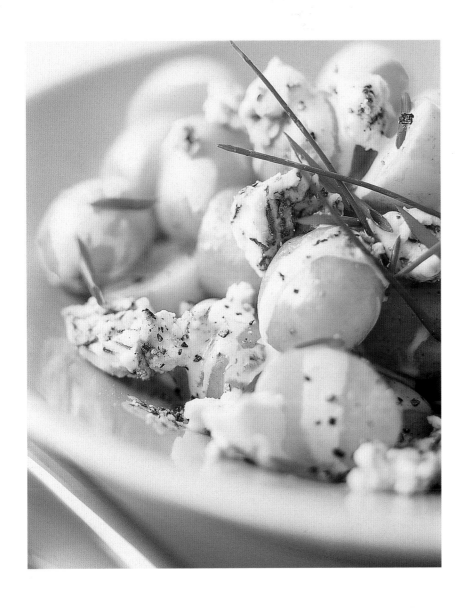

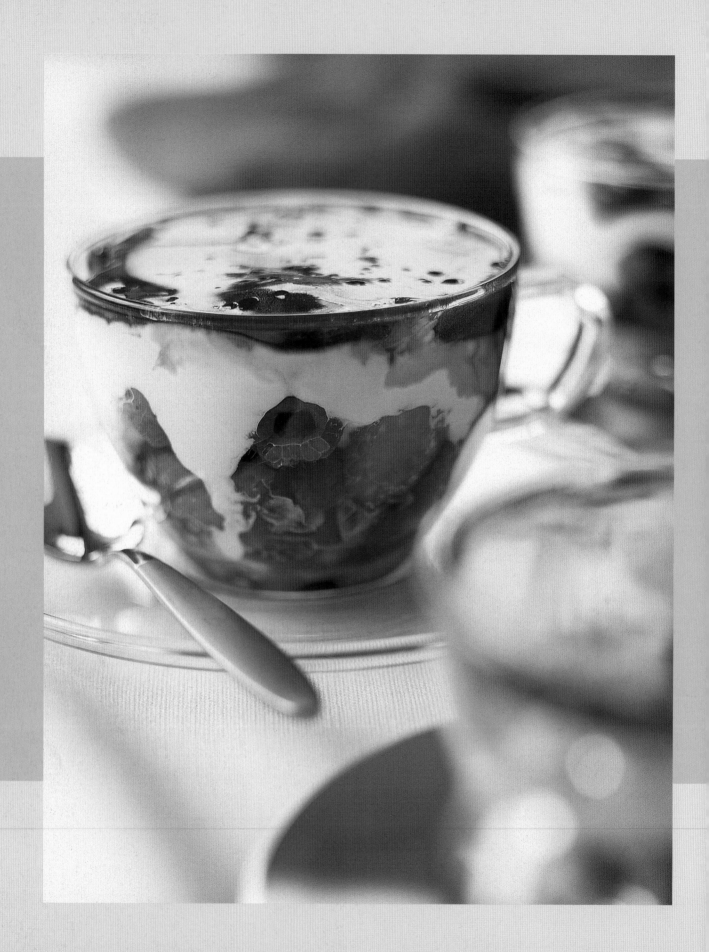

# 6 Puddings & Treats

Though we don't normally think of desserts as being nutritious, they can provide good quantities of vitamins and minerals. The recipes that follow incorporate carefully chosen, healthy ingredients, and all taste delicious.

# FUDGY NUT PIE

225 g ready-made shortcrust pastry

Flour, for dusting

75 g plain chocolate, broken into small pieces

50 g butter

175 g golden caster sugar

75 g soft light brown sugar

100 ml full-fat milk

75 g golden syrup

1 teaspoon vanilla essence

½ teaspoon salt

3 eggs

125 g mixed nuts, chopped

Icing sugar, for dusting

Serves 6

*This dessert is deliciously indulgent and is bound to be a hit with the whole family. Serve with vanilla ice cream or crème fraîche.*

1   Roll out the pastry on a lightly floured surface and use to line a 23 cm loose-bottomed, 4 cm deep, flan tin. Place on a baking sheet, cover and chill for 30 minutes. Preheat the oven to 200°C, gas mark 6.

2   Prick the pastry with a fork, then line with a large sheet of greaseproof paper and fill with baking beans. Bake for 10–15 minutes, then carefully remove the paper and the beans and return to the oven for a further 5 minutes, until the base is firm to the touch and lightly golden. Remove from the oven and set aside while making the filling.

3   To make the filling, melt the chocolate and butter in a large bowl over hot water. Remove from the heat and add the sugar, milk, golden syrup, vanilla essence, salt and eggs. Beat with a wooden spoon until smooth, then stir in the nuts.

4   Pour the filling into the pastry case and bake at 180°C, gas mark 4 for 45–55 minutes, until puffy and golden. Leave to cool. Dust with icing sugar to serve.

# SPICED APPLE & RAISIN PANCAKES

### FOR THE FILLING

50 g raisins

3 tablespoons dark rum

900 g Bramley apples, peeled, cored and sliced

5 tablespoons water

3–4 tablespoons caster sugar

Pinch of ground cinnamon

*A sweet treat that isn't loaded with fat or calories, these pancakes are delicious served on their own, or with a scoop of vanilla ice cream.*

1   To make the filling, place the raisins in a small bowl, pour over the rum and leave to stand for 30 minutes. Place the apples and water in a large pan, cover, and cook gently for about 10 minutes, stirring occasionally. Stir in the sugar, cinnamon and soaked raisins.

2   To make the pancakes, place the flour and salt in a large bowl. Add the egg and half the milk and mix for 1 minute until the mixture is bubbly – use an electric hand mixer if you have one. Stir in the rest of the milk. Pour the batter into a jug and leave to stand for 20 minutes.

3   Heat an 18 cm pancake pan. Add a little oil and, when it starts to smoke, pour in just enough batter to thinly coat the base of the pan. Cook over a moderate heat for about 1 minute or until the bottom is golden brown. Turn the pancake over and cook on the other side for another 30 seconds. Slide the pancake onto a plate, cover with foil, and keep warm in a low oven (150°C, gas mark 2) while you make the rest of the pancakes. Add extra oil to the pan as necessary.

4   Gently reheat the apple mixture. Spoon a little of the mixture into the middle of each pancake and roll. Serve with Greek yogurt.

### FOR THE PANCAKES

125 g plain flour, sieved

Pinch of salt

1 large egg

300 ml semi-skimmed milk

Sunflower oil, for frying

Greek yogurt, to serve

Serves 4 (makes 8 pancakes)

# RICH CHOCOLATE & FIG PUDDINGS WITH CHOCOLATE SAUCE

*The chocolate and figs complement each other perfectly to produce these wonderfully rich, fruity desserts. A generous spoonful of crème fraîche is a good accompaniment.*

1   Preheat the oven to 180°C, gas mark 4. Mix the figs and syrup together and divide the mixture between 6 buttered 150 ml dariole moulds.

2   Cream the butter and sugar together until light and fluffy, then beat in the eggs, a little at a time. Sift the flour, baking powder and cocoa powder together and fold into the egg mixture. Stir in the melted chocolate and breadcrumbs.

3   Spoon the mixture into the dariole moulds until they are two-thirds full. Cover with foil and place in a roasting tin containing enough hot water to come half-way up the moulds. Bake for 35–40 minutes, then leave to stand for 5 minutes.

4   Meanwhile, make the chocolate sauce. Place the chocolate and butter in a bowl over a saucepan of hot water and stir until melted. Add the milk and rum and stir for 1 minute.

5   Turn out the cake and sprinkle with chocolate shavings. Serve with the chocolate sauce poured over.

100 g ready-to-eat dried figs, chopped

4 tablespoons maple syrup

100 g unsalted butter, softened, plus extra for greasing

100 g light muscovado sugar

3 eggs, lightly beaten

75 g self-raising flour

1 teaspoon baking powder

1 tablespoon cocoa powder

100 g plain chocolate, melted

75 g fresh white breadcrumbs

Chocolate shavings, for sprinkling

### FOR THE CHOCOLATE SAUCE

125 g plain chocolate

25 g butter

1 tablespoon full-fat milk

1 tablespoon rum

Serves 6

# Dates Stuffed with Ricotta

50 g ricotta cheese

1 tablespoon icing sugar

6 fresh dates

15 g pistachio nuts, chopped

Serves 2

*This sweet treat makes a light dessert that is perfect for after a heavy meal. The cool, creamy ricotta cheese provides a delicious complement to the sweetness of the dates.*

1   Mix the ricotta and icing sugar together in a small bowl.

2   Make a lengthways cut in each date and remove the stone.

3   Spoon a little of the ricotta mixture into the centre of each date. Sprinkle over a few chopped pistachio nuts and serve.

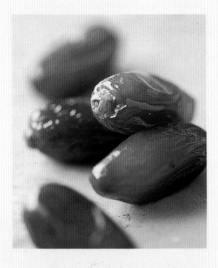

# Brandied Prunes with Greek Yogurt

225 g pitted ready-to-eat dried prunes

50 g large seedless raisins

150 ml cold tea

3 tablespoons brandy

8 tablespoons Greek yogurt

2 tablespoons icing sugar

6 brandy snaps, to serve

Serves 6

*Plump and succulent prunes make a light and tasty dessert. Prunes are a good source of fibre and provide useful amounts of calcium and iron.*

1   Place the prunes and raisins in a large bowl and pour over the tea and brandy. Cover and leave to soak for at least 6 hours, or preferably overnight.

2   When ready to serve, beat together the Greek yogurt and icing sugar. Spoon the brandied prunes into serving bowls and top each with a spoonful of the yogurt mixture and a brandy snap.

# LEMON & STRAWBERRY CHEESECAKE

*This fresh, lemony cheesecake makes a perfect dinner party dessert or a snack with morning coffee.*

1  To make the base, place the biscuits in a plastic bag, seal, then crush with a rolling pin to make fine crumbs. Melt the butter in a saucepan, then stir in the biscuit crumbs and demerara sugar. Press the mixture into the base and sides of a 20 cm loose-bottomed flan tin and chill until set.

2  To make the filling, place the lemon zest in a bowl. Add the cream cheese and condensed milk and beat until smooth. Very gradually beat in the lemon juice until the mixture is thick and creamy. In another bowl, whip the cream until it forms soft peaks, then fold into the cream cheese mixture.

3  Spoon the cheesecake mixture into the biscuit base and swirl the top with the back of a spoon. Arrange the strawberries cut-side down around the edge and chill for 1 hour.

4  For the strawberry sauce, put 225 g of the strawberries into a bowl and stir in the sugar and orange liqueur. Chill for 1 hour, then blend in a food processor or blender until smooth. Pass the purée through a fine nylon sieve to remove the seeds, then stir in the remaining strawberries and the orange zest.

5  To serve, remove the cheesecake from the tin and slice. Decorate with mint sprigs and serve with the strawberry sauce.

### LEMON & RASPBERRY CHEESECAKE
Replace the strawberries with raspberries in both the filling and the sauce.

## FOR THE CHEESECAKE BASE

225 g digestive biscuits

125 g butter

1 tablespoon demerara sugar

## FOR THE FILLING

Zest of 1 lemon

225 g full-fat cream cheese

215 g canned sweetened condensed milk

Juice of 3 lemons

140 ml double cream

125 g fresh strawberries, cut in half

## FOR THE STRAWBERRY SAUCE

450 g small ripe strawberries, cut into quarters

50 g caster sugar

2 tablespoons orange-flavoured liqueur

Zest of 1 orange

Fresh mint sprigs, to decorate

Serves 6–8

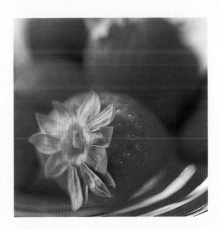

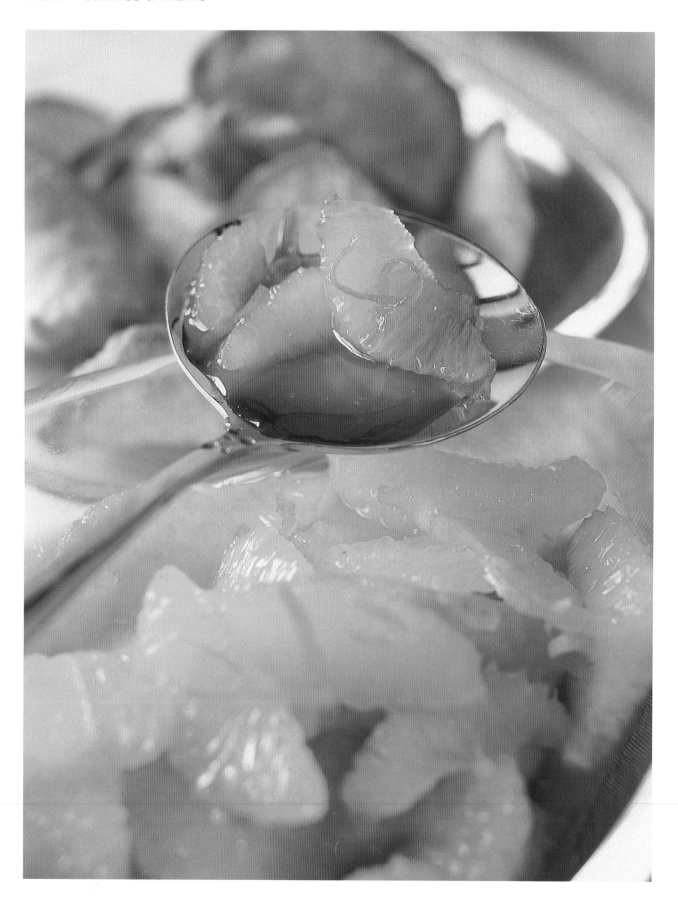

# CARAMEL ORANGES WITH ALMOND & SESAME SEED BISCUITS

*Oranges are a useful source of calcium and also provide plenty of other vitamins and minerals, especially vitamin C. These biscuits make a light, low-fat, tasty dessert.*

1   Remove the zest from 3 of the oranges and reserve. To peel the oranges, slice them all across the top and bottom to reveal the flesh, then remove the skin and pith in strips by slicing downwards, following the shape of the orange.

2   Working over a bowl, remove the orange segments by slicing carefully between each segment and its membrane. Reserve the juice in the bowl. Put the orange segments to one side.

3   To make the orange caramel, put the sugar in a heavy-based saucepan with 3 tablespoons of water. Heat gently until the sugar dissolves, then bring to a rapid boil until it turns a rich, golden colour.

4   Remove from the heat and carefully add the honey, the reserved orange juice and half the reserved orange zest. The caramel will form a blob on the bottom of the pan, so return to a gentle heat and dissolve in the juice. When the mixture is smooth, set aside to cool.

5   When cool, pour the caramel over the orange segments. Chill in the fridge until ready to serve.

6   Meanwhile, make the almond sesame biscuits. Preheat the oven to 220°C, gas mark 7. Whisk the egg whites until stiff, then add the sugar and whisk for 1 minute until the mixture is glossy. Using a metal spoon, fold in the flour, butter, sesame seeds, almonds and the reserved orange zest.

7   Put teaspoons of the mixture onto a baking tray lined with baking parchment, about 6 cm apart. Bake for 5–6 minutes until golden, then remove from the oven. While the biscuits are still warm, press with a rolling pin to curve them – they will harden in seconds. If the biscuits harden before shaping, return to the oven for a few minutes to soften.

8   To serve, remove the orange segments from the fridge and spoon into serving bowls. Serve with the almond sesame biscuits.

## FOR THE CARAMEL ORANGES

6 large oranges

200 g caster sugar

2 tablespoons runny honey

## FOR THE ALMOND SESAME BISCUITS

2 egg whites

125 g caster sugar

50 g plain flour, sifted

50 g butter, melted

2 tablespoons sesame seeds

50 g blanched almonds, chopped

Serves 6 (makes around 24 biscuits)

# MIXED BERRY BRULEE

*This classic dish is made healthier by replacing the cream with lower-fat Greek yogurt.*

125 g fresh blueberries

125 g fresh raspberries

125 g fresh strawberries, hulled and roughly chopped

Seeds and juice of 4 passion fruits

300 ml Greek yogurt

125 g soft brown sugar

Serves 4

1  Mix the blueberries, raspberries, strawberries and passion fruit seeds and juice together in a large bowl and divide between 4 ovenproof ramekins.

2  Spoon the yogurt over the fruit and chill for at least 2 hours.

3  Remove the ramekins from the fridge and sprinkle the sugar over the yogurt. Place under a hot grill until the sugar caramelises, then serve immediately.

# LEMON & PASSION FRUIT ROULADE

*Greek yogurt contains considerably less fat than double cream and about three times more calcium, helping to make this a healthier alternative to more traditional cream-filled desserts.*

## FOR THE MERINGUE

4 egg whites

225 g caster sugar

1 level tablespoon cornflour

2 teaspoons malt vinegar

1 teaspoon vanilla essence

## FOR THE FILLING

4 tablespoons lemon curd

Seeds and juice of 4 passion fruits

25 g flaked almonds, toasted, to decorate

Icing sugar, for dusting

200 ml Greek yogurt

Serves 6

1  Preheat the oven to 150°C, gas mark 2. Line the base and sides of a 31.5 × 21.5 cm Swiss roll tin with non-stick baking parchment.

2  With an electric whisk, beat the egg whites until they are frothy and have doubled in bulk, then gradually whisk in the sugar until the mixture is very thick and shiny. Whisk in the cornflour, vinegar and vanilla essence.

3  Spoon the mixture into the prepared tin and level the surface. Bake for 50 minutes, or until the surface is just firm.

4  Meanwhile, to make the filling, mix together the lemon curd and passion fruit seeds and juice.

5  Remove the meringue from the oven and allow to cool for 10 minutes. Turn out and carefully peel off the paper. Lightly dust a sheet of baking parchment with toasted almonds and icing sugar and place the meringue on the parchment. Spread the yogurt over the meringue, then drizzle the lemon and passion fruit mixture over the yogurt.

6  Using the parchment to help you, roll up the meringue from one of the long ends. Refrigerate for at least 30 minutes, or until ready to serve.

# APRICOT RISOTTO

*This dessert is a variation on traditional rice pudding – the fruity apricot coulis adds a healthy, modern twist.*

1  Place the canned apricots in a blender or food processor and purée until smooth. Set to one side. Place the milk and sugar in a saucepan and gently heat, stirring occasionally, until the milk reaches simmering point. Reduce the heat and allow the milk to simmer.

2  Melt the butter in a large saucepan, add the rice and cook, stirring, for 1–2 minutes. Add the chopped apricots and cook for 1–2 minutes.

3  Add a ladle of the warm milk and cook, stirring continuously, until the liquid is absorbed. Continue adding the milk in the same way until all the milk is used and the rice is tender – this will take about 20 minutes.

4  Stir the puréed apricots into the rice, then spoon into bowls and decorate with toasted almonds.

400 g can apricots in natural juice, drained

1 litre full-fat milk

2 tablespoons caster sugar

15 g butter

150 g arborio rice

100 g ready-to eat dried apricots, roughly chopped

2 tablespoons flaked almonds, toasted

Serves 4

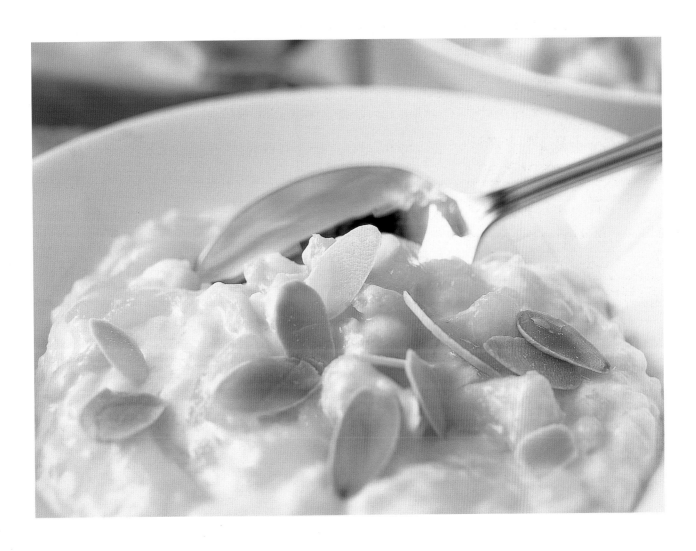

# FROZEN STRAWBERRY YOGURT

500 g strawberries, hulled and roughly chopped

3 tablespoons apple juice

2 tablespoons crème de cassis (optional)

4 tablespoons icing sugar

500 ml Greek yogurt

Fresh fruit, to decorate

Serves 4

*This is a healthy treat for a hot day. Although you can buy frozen yogurt in most supermarkets, if you have the time it is really worth making your own – once you've eaten home-made, shop-bought will never taste quite the same. The frozen yogurt can be stored for up to 2 weeks in the freezer.*

1  Place the strawberries in a saucepan. Add the apple juice and gently warm, stirring occasionally, until the strawberries become soft and pulpy.

2  Press the strawberries through a nylon sieve and collect their juice in a large bowl. Discard the seeds. Allow to cool completely, then beat in the crème de cassis (if using), icing sugar and yogurt.

3  Pour the mixture into an ice-cream machine and churn until it becomes thick and frozen. If you don't have an ice-cream machine, transfer the mixture to a shallow freezerproof container. Freeze for at least 1 hour, or until the mixture begins to set around the edges. Remove the container from the freezer and beat the mixture until smooth, then return to the freezer. Freeze for another 30 minutes then beat again. Repeat the freezing and beating process two more times.

4  Transfer the frozen yogurt from the freezer to the fridge 20 minutes before serving. Decorate with fresh fruit to serve.

# LEMON MASCARPONE ICE CREAM

500 g mascarpone cheese

1 tablespoon lemon juice

Zest of 2 lemons

125 g icing sugar

3 egg yolks

2 tablespoons orange-flavoured liqueur

Fresh berries, to serve

Serves 6

*This is an ideal dessert for a dinner party, especially when served with a selection of fresh summer berries. Remember that raw eggs are not suitable for the elderly, pregnant women, young children or people who have immune deficiency disease.*

1  Beat the mascarpone cheese, lemon juice and zest, icing sugar, egg yolks and orange-flavoured liqueur together in a large bowl, until smooth.

2  Freeze the mixture in an ice cream maker, if you have one, or in a freezerproof container. If you use a freezerproof container, beat the mixture at hourly intervals until the ice cream is frozen – this helps to prevent ice crystals forming and ensures an even-textured result.

3  Once frozen, remove the ice cream from the freezer and serve with fresh berries.

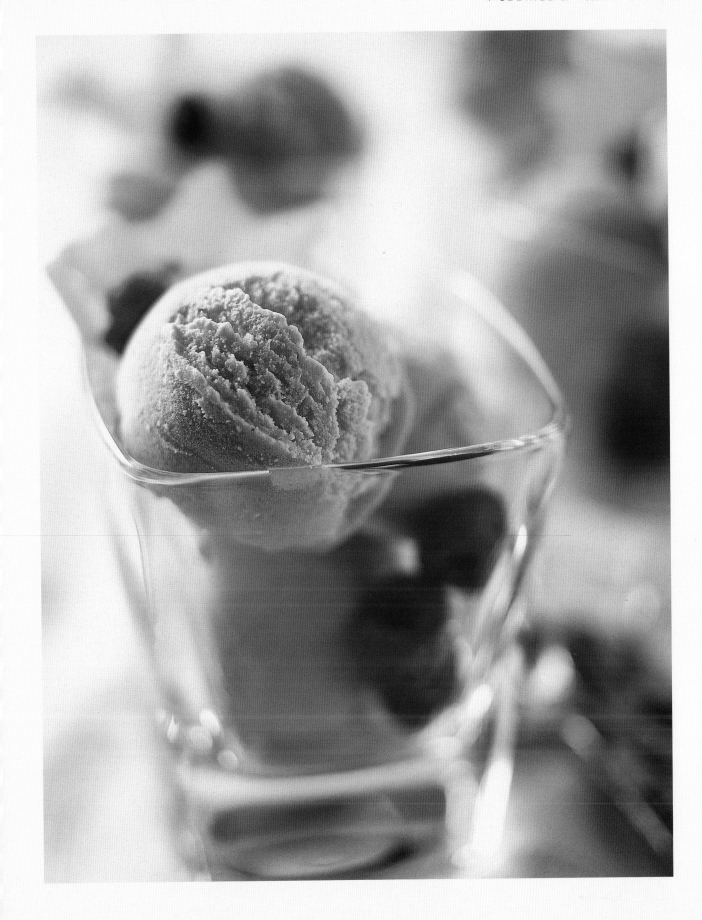

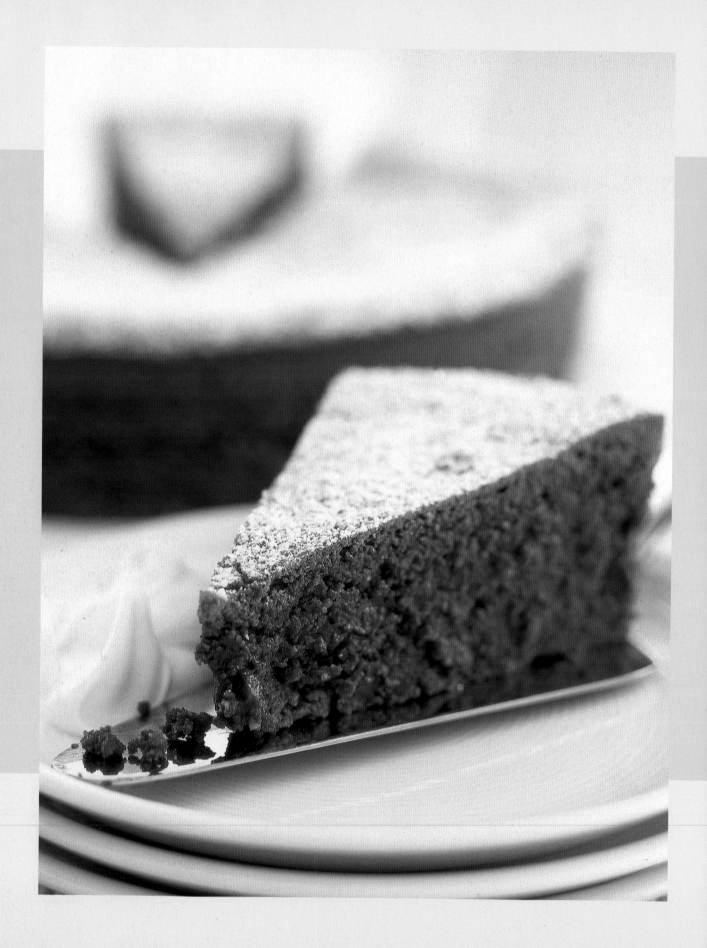

# 7 Home Bakes

This chapter offers a selection of savoury snacks, biscuits and cakes that make delicious treats at any time of day. The bakes feature ingredients such as cheese, nuts, seeds and fruit, which boost their calcium content, making them great for healthy bones.

# SUN-DRIED TOMATO & PARMESAN CORN BREAD SQUARES

*Serve this tasty bread with a bowl of steaming hot soup for a healthy and filling lunchtime snack.*

1 large egg, beaten

200 ml Greek yogurt

25 g butter, melted

150 g fine cornmeal

25 g flour

1 tablespoon baking powder

1 teaspoon fresh rosemary, chopped

½ teaspoon salt

50 g sun-dried tomatoes in oil, roughly chopped

125 g canned sweetcorn, drained

50 g Parmesan cheese, freshly grated

Makes 9 squares

1 Preheat the oven to 180°C, gas mark 4. Line the bottom of an 18 cm square tin, approximately 3 cm deep, with non-stick baking parchment.

2 Mix the egg, yogurt and melted butter together. Stir in the cornmeal, flour, baking powder, rosemary and salt. Add the sun-dried tomatoes, sweetcorn and Parmesan and mix until thoroughly combined.

3 Turn the mixture into the prepared tin and bake for 30–40 minutes, or until a skewer inserted into the centre of the loaf comes out clean.

4 Allow to cool in the tin for 10 minutes then turn out onto a cooling rack. When the bread is completely cold, cut into squares.

# CHEESE & WATERCRESS SCONES

*Light and easy to make, these scones make a delicious daytime snack. Watercress is an excellent source of vitamin C and vitamin E and provides substantial amounts of folic acid, niacin and vitamin B6.*

300 g self-raising white flour, sieved

1 teaspoon baking powder

50 g butter, diced

125 g watercress, chopped with stalks removed

125 g Gruyère cheese, grated

Salt and pepper, to taste

100 ml semi-skimmed milk, plus extra to glaze

Flour, for dusting

Makes 8 scones

1 Preheat the oven to 220°C, gas mark 7. Place the flour and baking powder in a large bowl. Rub in the butter with your fingertips, until the mixture resembles fine breadcrumbs.

2 Stir in the watercress, 75 g of the cheese and the seasoning. Add the milk and stir to form a smooth, soft dough.

3 Turn the dough out on to a well-floured surface and roll out to 2 cm thick. Using a 7.5 cm round cutter, cut out the scones. Press the trimmings together, re-roll and cut out more scones, until all the dough has been used.

4 Place the scones on a greased baking sheet. Brush the tops with milk, sprinkle over the remaining cheese and bake for 10–15 minutes, or until golden brown. Transfer to a wire rack to cool.

# PARMESAN & HERB TWISTS

*These tasty little snacks are the perfect accompaniment for a glass of chilled white wine, and can also be served with dips or soups. They will keep for up to one week in an air-tight container.*

1  Preheat the oven to 220°C, gas mark 7. Dust the work surface and rolling pin with a little flour. Roll out the pastry until it is very thin, then trim into a neat rectangle or square. Cut in half.

2  Sprinkle one half of the pastry with an even layer of Parmesan cheese, chopped rosemary and thyme. Dampen the edges, then carefully place the other piece of pastry on top and gently press down.

3  Using a kitchen knife, cut the Parmesan and herb pastry into strips. Twist each strip around a few times, then place on a baking sheet. Press the ends of the twists down so that they stick to the baking sheet – this stops them unwinding as they cook.

4  Bake the twists for about 10–12 minutes, or until golden brown, then remove the baking sheet from the oven. Leave them on the baking sheet for 5 minutes, then place on a wire rack to cool.

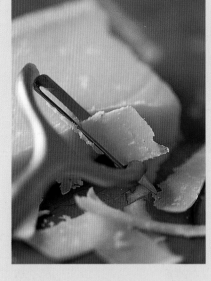

Plain flour, for dusting

500 g ready-made puff pastry

25 g Parmesan cheese, grated

2 tablespoons fresh rosemary, chopped

1 tablespoon fresh thyme leaves, chopped

Makes about 24 twists

## PESTO & PARMESAN TWISTS

Replace the rosemary and thyme with 3 tablespoons of green pesto (see recipe page 48). Spread the pesto over one half of the pastry and sprinkle with Parmesan. Then follow steps 3 and 4 as above.

# SODA BREAD

*This classic Irish recipe is extremely healthy and couldn't be easier to make. It's delicious served warm with slices of mature cheddar cheese.*

350 g plain wholemeal flour

125 g pinhead oatmeal

2 teaspoons bicarbonate of soda

1 teaspoon salt

1 teaspoon sugar

300 ml buttermilk

3–4 tablespoons semi-skimmed milk

Makes 1 loaf

1 Preheat the oven to 200°C, gas mark 6. Place the flour, oatmeal, bicarbonate of soda, salt and sugar in a large bowl. Make a well in the centre and gradually beat in the buttermilk and enough milk to form a soft dough.

2 Knead the dough for 5 minutes, or until smooth. Shape into a round about 20 cm in diameter. Using a sharp knife, cut a deep cross on the top of the dough. Place on a non-stick baking tray.

3 Bake for 30–40 minutes or until the bread sounds hollow when tapped on the bottom. Serve warm or leave to cool on a wire rack.

# BANANA & PUMPKIN LOAF

*This moist fruity loaf is delicious served plain, but for a special treat, try adding the mascarpone topping on page 123.*

100 ml sunflower oil, plus extra for greasing

125 g self-raising flour

75 g self-raising wholemeal flour

½ teaspoon bicarbonate of soda

1 teaspoon ground cinnamon

100 g soft brown sugar

4 tablespoons buttermilk or plain yogurt

2 eggs, beaten

250 g pumpkin, coarsely grated

1 medium banana, mashed

125 g sultanas

Makes 1 loaf

1 Preheat the oven to 180°C, gas mark 4. Lightly grease and line the base of a 900 g loaf tin with non-stick baking parchment.

2 Sift the flours, bicarbonate of soda and cinnamon into a large bowl. Stir in the sugar. Place the oil, buttermilk or yogurt and eggs in a separate bowl and whisk to combine. Pour the liquid into the flour and beat with an electric whisk for 1 minute.

3 Stir in the pumpkin, banana and sultanas and transfer the mixture to the prepared tin. Bake for 1 hour, or until a skewer inserted into the middle comes out clean. Allow to cool in the tin for 5–10 minutes, then carefully transfer to a wire rack to cool completely.

# SESAME OAT CRISPS

*Sesame seeds are a good source of calcium and vitamin E and give these biscuits a delicious nutty flavour.*

1 Preheat the oven to 180°C, gas mark 4. Lightly grease 2 baking sheets.

2 Place the butter, syrup and sugar in a large saucepan. Heat the mixture gently, stirring occasionally, until the butter melts and the sugar dissolves.

3 Stir in the porridge oats, sesame seeds and flour and mix well.

4 Dissolve the bicarbonate of soda in 1 teaspoon of hot water and stir into the mixture.

5 Allow the mixture to cool slightly, then roll into walnut-sized balls. Place on the prepared baking sheets, allowing plenty of space for the mixture to spread as it bakes (you may need to cook the crisps in batches). Bake for 15 minutes, or until evenly browned.

6 Remove the crisps from the oven and leave on the baking sheets to cool slightly. Using a palette knife, transfer to a wire rack to cool completely.

125 g butter, plus extra for greasing

1 heaped tablespoon golden syrup

125 g demerara sugar

75 g porridge oats

50 g sesame seeds

125 g plain white flour

1 teaspoon bicarbonate of soda

Makes about 26 crisps

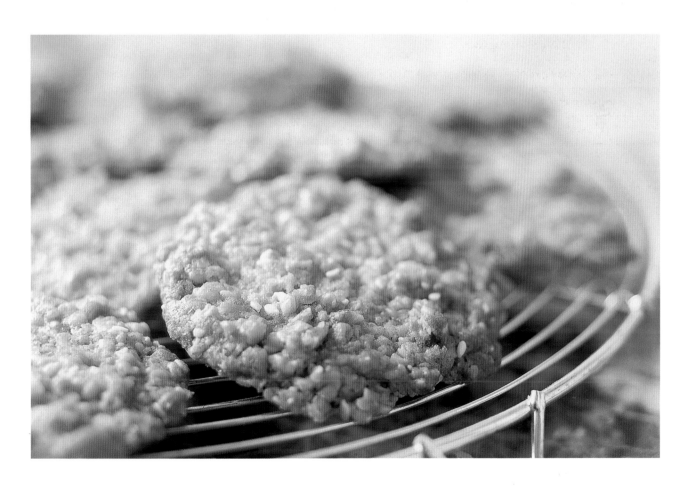

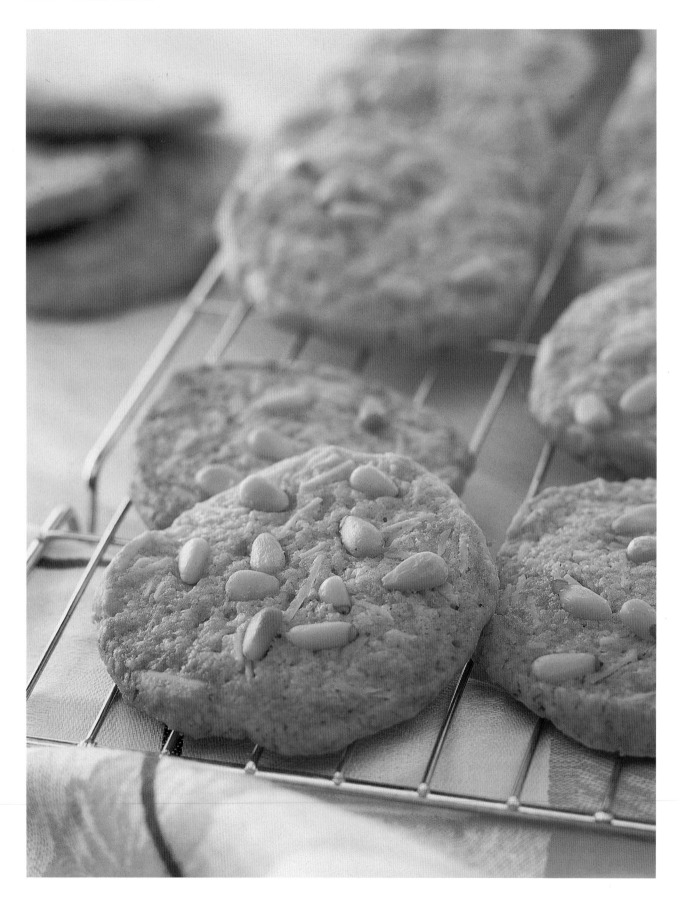

# ALMOND & PINE NUT COOKIES

*Nuts are a good source of B vitamins and minerals, making
these cookies a healthy and tasty treat.*

1  Preheat the oven to 190°C, gas mark 5. Lightly grease 2 baking sheets.

2  Sift the flour and bicarbonate of soda into a bowl. Add the butter and rub
it in with your fingertips until the mixture resembles fine breadcrumbs.
Add the sugar and almonds, then stir in the egg, orange zest and almond
extract and mix to a dough, adding a little milk if necessary.

3  Turn out onto a lightly floured surface and shape into a cylinder about
23 cm long. Cut into thin slices and place on the baking sheets. Sprinkle
over the pine nuts, pressing them down lightly with your fingertips.

4  Bake the cookies for 8–10 minutes until pale golden (you may need to cook
them in batches). Allow to cool slightly before lifting them onto a wire
rack, then leave to cool completely.

200 g plain flour, plus extra for dusting

½ teaspoon bicarbonate of soda

125 g butter, diced

125 g golden caster sugar

75 g flaked almonds, roughly chopped

1 egg, lightly beaten

Zest of 1 orange

Few drops almond extract

2 tablespoons milk

50 g pine nuts, finely chopped

Makes 27 cookies

APRICOT & PINE NUT COOKIES
Replace the almonds with 50 g finely chopped, ready-to-eat dried apricots.
Follow the recipe as above, omitting the almond extract.

# APRICOT & ORANGE MUFFINS

175 g plain white flour

2 teaspoons baking powder

Pinch salt

25 g golden caster sugar

2 tablespoons runny honey

1 egg

75 ml orange juice

75 ml full-fat milk

50 g butter, melted and cooled

50 g ready-to-eat dried apricots, chopped

Makes 6 muffins

*These light-as-air muffins are studded with chewy apricots and orange zest. For a treat, they can also be served at breakfast.*

1 Preheat the oven to 200°C, gas mark 6. Line 6 deep muffin tins with paper cases.

2 Sieve the flour, baking powder and salt into a large bowl. In another large bowl, mix together the sugar, honey, egg, orange juice, milk and cooled butter. Sieve the dry ingredients into the egg mixture and fold in gently with a metal spoon. Do not beat or whisk the mixture.

3 Lightly fold in the chopped apricots. then divide the mixture equally between the paper cases. Bake for 15 minutes, or until well-risen and golden brown. A skewer inserted into the centre of the muffins should come out clean. Leave in the tin for a few minutes, then transfer to a wire rack to cool. Serve warm or cold.

# CITRUS YOGURT CAKE

200 ml natural yogurt

225 g golden caster sugar

125 g butter, melted, plus extra for greasing

3 eggs

Zest of ½ lemon, grated

Zest of ½ orange, grated

Zest of 1 lime, grated

350 g plain flour

FOR THE MASCARPONE CREAM

250 g mascarpone cheese

1 tablespoon orange thin-cut marmalade

Icing sugar, for dusting

Serves 8

*This moist citrus cake is made with natural yogurt and served with a lovely mascarpone cream. Another way to serve this cake is to split it in half and sandwich the two halves together with the mascarpone cream, then dredge the top with icing sugar.*

1 Preheat the oven to 180°C, gas mark 4. Lightly grease a 20 cm loose bottomed shallow cake tin and line the base with greaseproof paper.

2 In a large bowl, whisk together the yogurt, sugar, melted butter, eggs, lemon and orange and lime zest. Beat in the flour until well mixed.

3 Pour the cake mixture into the prepared tin and bake in the centre of the oven for 45–50 minutes, or until a skewer inserted into the centre of the cake comes out clean. Leave to cool for 10 minutes, then transfer to a cake rack to cool completely.

4 Meanwhile, beat the mascarpone with the marmalade. Cover and chill until ready to use.

5 Dust the top of the cake with icing sugar. Cut into wedges and serve with a spoonful of the mascarpone cream.

# LEMON & POPPY SEED DRIZZLE LOAF CAKE

*Poppy seeds are a useful source of calcium, particularly for people on dairy-free diets. This cake is good on its own or with a spoonful of crème fraîche or Greek yogurt.*

1   Preheat the oven to 180°C, gas mark 4. Grease and line a 1.4 litre loaf tin.

2   Place the butter or margarine, sugar, eggs, flour, baking powder, salt, lemon zest and juice into a food processor and process until smooth. Fold in the poppy seeds.

3   Spoon the mixture into the prepared tin and level the surface. Bake for 50–55 minutes, or until well-risen and firm to the touch. Turn out and cool on a wire rack.

4   For the topping, mix the icing sugar with enough lemon juice to form a smooth consistency. Drizzle over the top of the cake and decorate with the shredded candied lemon peel.

## FOR THE CAKE

225 g butter or margarine

175 g golden caster sugar

3 eggs

350 g self-raising wholemeal flour

1 teaspoon baking powder

Pinch salt

Zest and juice of 2 large lemons

50 g poppy seeds

## FOR THE TOPPING

75 g icing sugar

2–3 teaspoons lemon juice

Candied lemon peel, shredded, to decorate

Makes 12 slices

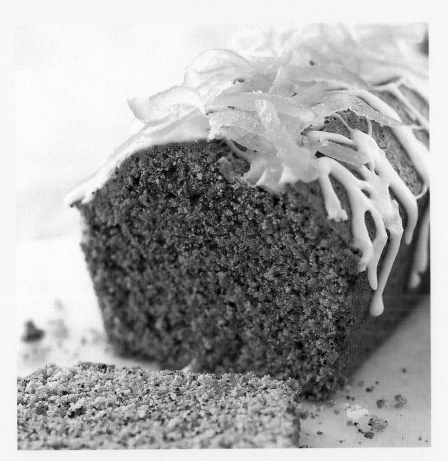

# RICH CHOCOLATE CAKE

200 g dark chocolate (about 70 per cent cocoa solid)

2 teaspoons instant coffee granules

200 g unsalted butter, softened

200 g caster sugar

4 eggs, separated

150 g ground almonds

75 g cornflour

Icing sugar, for dusting

Crème fraîche, to serve

Serves 10

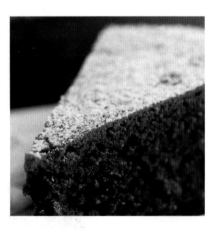

*This moist, rich chocolate cake not only tastes fantastic but if you serve it with Greek yogurt or reduced-fat crème fraîche you can boost the calcium content.*

1  Preheat the oven to 180°C, gas mark 4. Lightly grease a 20 cm loose bottomed shallow cake tin and line the base with greaseproof paper.

2  Place the chocolate and coffee in a bowl over a pan of simmering water and melt. In a large bowl, cream the butter and sugar until pale and fluffy. Beat in the eggs yolks, one at a time, then stir in the chocolate and coffee mixture, almonds and cornflour.

3  In a large clean bowl, whisk the egg whites until they form soft peaks. Fold a quarter of the whisked egg whites into the chocolate mixture to loosen it, then gradually fold in the remainder. Pour the mixture into the prepared tin and bake for 50–60 minutes, or until it springs back when touched. Cover the cake with greaseproof paper after 50 minutes. Allow to cool completely before carefully removing it from the tin.

4  Cut the cake into wedges, dust with a little icing sugar and serve with crème fraîche, if liked.

# CARROT CAKE WITH MASCARPONE TOPPING

FOR THE CARROT CAKE

Butter, for greasing

Flour, for dusting

225 g unsalted butter or margarine, softened

225 g golden caster sugar

175 g self-raising white flour

1 teaspoon baking powder

½ teaspoon ground allspice

4 eggs

Zest of 1 large orange

*This cake is guaranteed to be a hit with both children and adults. The mascarpone cheese makes a deliciously rich and creamy frosting.*

1  Preheat the oven to 180°C, gas mark 4. Grease two 20 cm sandwich tins. Dust the sides of the tins with flour and shake out the excess.

2  Cream the butter or margarine and sugar together in a bowl until pale and fluffy. Sift the flour, baking powder and allspice into the bowl. Add the eggs, orange rind and juice and ground almonds and beat well, then stir in the walnuts and the carrots.

3  Divide the mixture equally between the two tins and level the surface. Bake for 35–40 minutes until the cakes have risen and are firm to the touch. Leave in the tins for 5 minutes, then transfer to a wire rack to cool.

4 For the topping, beat the mascarpone cheese and icing sugar together in a bowl until smooth. Use half of the mixture to sandwich the cake together, then spread the remaining mixture over the top of the cake. Arrange the walnut halves around the edge of the cake to decorate.

### ORANGE MASCARPONE TOPPING

Beat together 500 g mascarpone cheese with 1 teaspoon orange zest, 2 tablespoons orange juice and 2 tablespoons icing sugar. Use to sandwich the cake together and spread the remainder over the top of the cake. Decorate with walnuts and orange zest.

1 tablespoon orange juice

50 g ground almonds

200 g carrots, finely grated

125 g walnuts, coarsely chopped

### FOR THE MASCARPONE TOPPING

500 g mascarpone cheese

2 tablespoons icing sugar

50 g walnut halves, to decorate

Serves 8–10

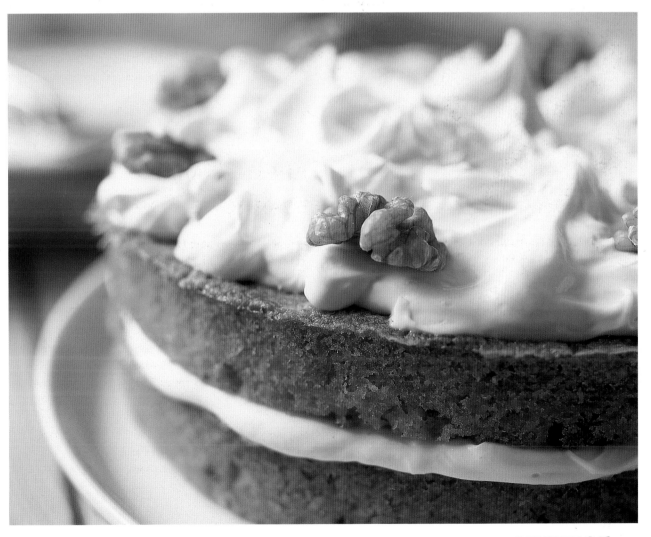

# Nutritional Analysis

The nutritional information for each recipe refers to a single serving, unless otherwise stated. Optional ingredients are not included. The figures are intended as a guide only. If salt is given in a measured amount in the recipe, it has been included in the analysis; if the recipe suggests adding a pinch of salt or seasoning to taste, salt has not been included.

p.106 Sweet Fruit Porridge
calories 235; KJ 996; protein 6g;
fat 4g; saturated fat 1g; fibre 3g;
sodium 50mg; calcium 75mg

p.106 Apple & Blueberry
Muesli
calories 460–306; KJ 1944–1296;
protein 15–10g; fat 13–9g;
saturated fat 1g; fibre 7.5–5g;
sodium 127–85mg;
calcium 330–220mg

p.107 Spiced Fruit Compote
calories 340; KJ 1452; protein
7g; fat 9g; saturated fat 3g;
fibre 5g; sodium 293mg;
calcium 143mg

p.108 Dried Fruit Spread
calories 40; KJ 152; protein 1g;
fat 0g; saturated fat 0g;
fibre 1g; sodium 6mg;
calcium 25mg

p.108 Bagels with Raspberries
& Ricotta
calories 300; KJ 1220;
protein 12g; fat 6g;
saturated fat 3g; fibre 3g;
sodium 40mg;
calcium 100mg

p.108 Banana & Almond
Smoothie
calories 320; KJ 1350;
protein 13g; fat 15g;
saturated fat 4g; fibre 3g;
sodium 128mg;
calcium 325mg

p.109 Apricot & Orange
Smoothie
calories 170; KJ 727; protein 3g;
fat 1g; saturated fat 0g;
fibre 4g; sodium 29mg;
calcium 65mg

p.109 Strawberry Smoothie
calories 100; KJ 410; protein 6g;
fat 3g; saturated fat 0.5g;
fibre 2g; sodium 60mg;
calcium 70mg

p.111 Cheesy Scrambled Eggs
calories 300; KJ 1270;
protein 22g; fat 23g;
saturated fat 10g; fibre 0g;
sodium 365mg;
calcium 268mg

p.111 Smoked Haddock
Omelette
calories 390; KJ 1629;
protein 36g; fat 27g;
saturated fat 12g; fibre 0g;
sodium 1136mg;
calcium 317mg

p.112 Soft Eggs with Soured
Cream & Smoked Salmon
calories 310; KJ 1295;
protein 19g; fat 18g;
saturated fat 8g; fibre 1g;
sodium 779mg;
calcium 113mg

p.113 Smoked Haddock &
Sweetcorn Fritters
calories 244; KJ 1036;
protein 17g; fat 5g;
saturated fat 1g; fibre 3g;
sodium 733mg;
calcium 128mg

p.113 Stuffed Portobello
Mushrooms
calories 400; KJ 1199;
protein 24g; fat 11g;
saturated fat 3g; fibre 4.5g;
sodium 1199mg;
calcium 250mg

p.116 Broccoli & Stilton Soup
calories 275; KJ 1148;
protein 16g; fat 16g;
saturated fat 8g; fibre 4g;
sodium 525mg;
calcium 265mg

p.117 Moroccan Spiced
Chickpea Soup
calories 210; KJ 876;
protein 10g; fat 9g;
saturated fat 1g; fibre 6g;
sodium 440mg; calcium 90mg

p.117 Roasted Pepper Soup
with Feta & Basil
calories 140; KJ 580; protein 5g;
fat 8g; saturated fat 3g;
fibre 3g; sodium 392mg;
calcium 90mg

p.119 French Onion Soup
calories 370; KJ 1547;
protein 13g; fat 18g;
saturated fat 10g; fibre 3g;
sodium 869mg; calcium 288mg

p.119 Garden Pea &
Watercress Soup
calories 380; KJ 1605;
protein 12g; fat 27g;
saturated fat 7g;
fibre 7g; sodium 545mg;
calcium 118mg

p.120 Smoked Haddock &
Sweetcorn Chowder
calories 390; KJ 1638;
protein 35g; fat 9g;
saturated fat 5g; fibre 3g;
sodium 1865mg;
calcium 205mg

p.120 Baked Ricotta with
Roasted Vine Tomatoes
calories 350; KJ 14560;
protein 24g; fat 26g;
saturated fat 14g; fibre 1g;
sodium 484mg;
calcium 578mg

p.121 Mushroom & Goat's
Cheese in Aubergine Parcels
calories 260; KJ 1062;
protein 11g; fat 22g;
saturated fat 8g; fibre 4g;
sodium 301mg; calcium 144mg

p.122 Cherry Tomato & Goat's
Cheese Tartlets
calories 440; KJ 1838;
protein 13g; fat 32g;
saturated fat 10g; fibre 0.5g;
sodium 398mg;
calcium 200mg

p.122 Tomato & Mozzarella
Salad
calories 390; KJ 1622;
protein 20g; fat 33g;
saturated fat 12g; fibre 1.5g;
sodium 471mg;
calcium 453mg

p.123 Watercress, Pear &
Roquefort Salad
calories 425; KJ 1763;
protein 14g; fat 37g;
saturated fat 13g; fibre 3g;
sodium 857mg;
calcium 367mg

p.123 Avocado & Smoked
Salmon Rolls
calories 350; KJ 1476;
protein 25g; fat 27g;
saturated fat 10g;
fibre 2g; sodium 1473mg;
calcium 140mg

p.124 Roasted Red Pepper Dip
calories 135–90; KJ 570–380;
protein 18–12g; fat 1–4.5g;
saturated fat 0g; fibre 2–1g;
sodium 188–125mg;
calcium 150–100mg

p.124 Tzatziki
calories 125–83; KJ 512–341;
protein 7–5g; fat 9–6g;
saturated fat 5–3.5g; fibre 0.5g;
sodium 74–50mg;
calcium 166–111mg

p.124 Creamy Guacamole
calories 200; KJ 892; protein 3g;
fat 21g; saturated fat 5g;
fibre 4g; sodium 21mg;
calcium 40mg

p.128 Humous
calories 275; KJ 1144;
protein 9g; fat 21g;
saturated fat 3g; fibre 5g;
sodium 196mg;
calcium 140mg

p.128 Red Pepper Humous
calories 280; KJ 1184; protein
10g; fat 19g; saturated fat 3g;
fibre 6g; sodium 196mg;
calcium 122mg

p.129 Falafel with Salad in Pitta
calories 485; KJ 2050; protein 20g; fat 12g; saturated fat 1g; fibre 6g; sodium 905mg; calcium 205mg

p.130 Quick Ciabatta Pizza
calories 300; KJ 1241; protein 11g; fat 15g; saturated fat 5g; fibre 2g; sodium 440mg; calcium 130mg

p.130 Croque Monsieur
calories 555; KJ 2341; protein 23g; fat 36g; saturated fat 19g; fibre 1g; sodium 1012mg; calcium 554mg

p.132 Peppered Smoked Mackerel Spread
calories 342; KJ 1419; protein 19g; fat 29g; saturated fat 9g; fibre 0g; sodium 751mg; calcium 110mg

p.132 Chcken Tikka Salad
calories 290; KJ 1205; protein 29g; fat 18g; saturated fat 4g; fibre 1g; sodium 177mg; calcium 70mg

p.133 Chicken Caesar Salad with Parmesan Crisps
calories 425; KJ 1775; protein 38g; fat 23g; saturated fat 6g; fibre 1g; sodium 593mg; calcium 280mg

p.134 Feta Omelette with Rocket & Red Pepper
calories 500; KJ 2095; protein 28g; fat 41g; saturated fat 19g; fibre 1.5g; sodium 1315mg; calcium 356mg

p.134 Twice Baked Goat's Cheese Soufflé
calories 210; KJ 875; protein 9g; fat 16g; saturated fat 10g; fibre 0g; sodium 343mg; calcium 225mg

p.136 Spinach & Roquefort Pancakes
calories 430; KJ 1796; protein 22g; fat 25g; saturated fat 13g; fibre 4g; sodium 1294mg; calcium 654mg

p.136 Cajun Cheese Potato Skins with Tomato & Red Onion Salad
calories 300; KJ 1271; protein 12g; fat 14g; saturated fat 7g; fibre 2g; sodium 223mg; calcium 235mg

p.138 Bacon & Ricotta Tart
calories 400; KJ 1676; protein 18g; fat 20g; saturated fat 10g; fibre 2g; sodium 1255mg; calcium 229mg

p.139 Sweet Potato with Cottage Cheese & Crispy Bacon
calories 390; KJ 1652; protein 27g; fat 8g; saturated fat 4g; fibre 6g; sodium 1415mg; calcium 138mg

p.139 Spinach & Potato Cake
calories 420; KJ 1750; protein 18g; fat 24g; saturated fat 13g; fibre 4g; sodium 330mg; calcium 366g

p.142 Brie-stuffed Chicken with Creamy Pesto
calories 460; KJ 1931; protein 47g; fat 28g; saturated fat 13g; fibre 0g; sodium 937mg; calcium 300mg

p.143 Chicken & Wild Mushroom Stroganoff
calories 380; KJ 1568; protein 35g; fat 22g; saturated fat 10g; fibre 2g; sodium 388mg; calcium 27mg

p.143 Garlic Chicken in Yogurt
calories 440; KJ 1813; protein 29g; fat 34g; saturated fat 8g; fibre 2g; sodium 173mg; calcium 200mg

p.144 Coronation Chicken Salad
calories 760–506; KJ 3158–2105; protein 40–27g; fat 52–35g; saturated fat 15–10g; fibre 3–2g; sodium 565–376mg; calcium 115–77mg

p 145 Chicken & Sesame Bites
calories 300; KJ 1248; protein 23g; fat 17g; saturated fat 3g; fibre 2g; sodium 228mg; calcium 166mg

p.145 Quick Turkey Cassoulet
calories 560; KJ 2374; protein 58g; fat 15g; saturated fat 5g; fibre 12g; sodium 2318mg; calcium 336mg

p.146 Pork Stuffed with Apricots & Pine Nuts
calories 555–370; KJ 2320–1547; protein 53–35g; fat 29–19g; saturated fat 8–5g; fibre 2–1g; sodium 525–350mg; calcium 85–57mg

p.148 Pork with Pak Choi & Black Bean Sauce
calories 540; KJ 2273; protein 37g; fat 22g; saturated fat 5g; fibre 5g; sodium 1785mg; calcium 190mg

p.148 Pork Escalopes with Celeriac Cream Mash
calories 5116; KJ 2153; protein 31g; fat 29g; saturated fat 6g; fibre 6g; sodium 348mg; calcium 88mg

p.150 Polenta with Bacon & Mushrooms
calories 480; KJ 2000; protein 32g; fat 24g; saturated fat 11g; fibre 2g; sodium 1622mg; calcium 431mg

p.151 Broccoli & Smoked Ham Tagliatelle
calories 850; KJ 3557; protein 33g; fat 48g; saturated fat 29g; fibre 9g; sodium 1033mg; calcium 369mg

p.152 Skewered Lamb with Tomato, Chilli & Yogurt Marinade
calories 600; KJ 2500; protein 43g; fat 24g; saturated fat 8g; fibre 0g; sodium 275mg; calcium 75mg

p.153 Garlic & Cumin Roast Lamb with Chickpea & Apricot Salsa
calories 460; KJ 1919; protein 42g; fat 22g; saturated fat 8g; fibre 5g; sodium 334mg; calcium 70mg

p.154 Moroccan Lamb with Chickpea & Apricots
calories 440; KJ 1841; protein 32g; fat 15g; saturated fat 5g; fibre 6g; sodium 492mg; calcium 90mg

p.155 Moussaka
calories 540; KJ 2241; protein 43g; fat 31g; saturated fat 14g; fibre 4g; sodium 460mg; calcium 424mg

p.156 Shepherd's Pie
calories 510; KJ 2142; protein 35g; fat 23g; saturated fat 12g; fibre 5g; sodium 344mg; calcium 210mg

p.156 Blue Cheese & Walnut Steaks
calories 480; KJ 2000; protein 45g; fat 33g; saturated fat 14g; fibre 0g; sodium 488mg; calcium 125mg

p.157 Meatballs with Mozzarella & Tomato Sauce
calories 470; KJ 1964; protein 38g; fat 24g; saturated fat 10g; fibre 2g; sodium 505mg; calcium 271mg

p.159 Minced Beef with Polenta Topping
calories 630; KJ 2612; protein 39g; fat 34g; saturated fat 12g; fibre 3g; sodium 666mg; calcium 311mg

p.160 Salmon Fish Cakes
calories 540; KJ 2260; protein 29g; fat 27g; saturated fat 4g; fibre 12g; sodium 850mg; calcium 367mg

p.160 Salmon & Leek Lasagne
calories 590; KJ 2454; protein 37g; fat 34g; saturated fat 18g; fibre 2g; sodium 744mg; calcium 785mg

p.161 Smoked Salmon & Dill Quiche
calories 500; KJ 2090; protein 13g; fat 41g; saturated fat 21g; fibre 1g; sodium 718mg; calcium 140mg

p.162 Quick Salmon Kedgeree
calories 420; KJ 1741; protein 23g; fat 16g; saturated fat 6g; fibre 0g; sodium 303mg; calcium 206mg

p.162 Salmon with a Crumb Crust
calories 380; KJ 1590; protein 30g; fat 25g; carbohydrate 10g; fibre 0g; sodium 382mg; calcium 200mg

p.163 Cod & Broccoli Cheese Pie
calories 894; KJ 3712; protein 39g; fat 65g; saturated fat 41g; fibre 4g; sodium 617mg; calcium 394mg

p.164 Cod Baked in Yogurt
calories 160; KJ 680; protein 34g; fat 1.5g; saturated fat 0g; fibre 0g; sodium 258mg; calcium 87mg

p.164 Poached Haddock with Spinach & Poached Egg
calories 270; KJ 1147; protein 42g; fat 10g; saturated fat 3g; fibre 3g; sodium 1423mg; calcium 350mg

p.165 Fish Pie with Rosti Topping
calories 615; KJ 2552; protein 22g; fat 46g; saturated fat 28g; fibre 3g; sodium 891mg; calcium 123mg

p.165 Deep-fried Whitebait
calories 550; KJ 2299; protein 16g; fat 52g; saturated fat 6g; fibre 0g; sodium 278mg; calcium 711mg

p.166 Monkfish Kebabs with Roasted Vegetables & Pesto
calories 480; KJ 2000; protein 31g; fat 35g; saturated fat 8g; fibre 4g; sodium 523mg; calcium 240mg

p.167 Griddled Swordfish with Salsa Verde
calories 330; KJ 1358; protein 36g; fat 23g; saturated fat 4g; fibre 0g; sodium 365mg; calcium 45mg

p.168 Prawn & Spinach Roulade
calories 400; KJ 1636; protein 15g; fat 33g; saturated fat 19g; fibre 1g; sodium 895mg; calcium 218mg

p.168 Penne with Prawns & Asparagus
calories 680; KJ 2864; protein 42g; fat 33g; saturated fat 8g; fibre 3g; sodium 1844mg; calcium 456mg

p.170 Warm Lentil & Feta Salad
calories 404; KJ 1691; protein 22g; fat 22g; saturated fat 9g; fibre 6g; sodium 734mg; calcium 225mg

p.171 Spiced Spinach Lentil & Feta Filo Pie
calories 481; KJ 2000; protein 22g; fat 11g; saturated fat 5g; fibre 6g; sodium 682mg; calcium 306mg

p.172 Cheese & Leek Sausages
calories 372; KJ 1552; protein 14g; fat 24g; saturated fat 8g; fibre 1g; sodium 405mg; calcium 255mg

p.172 Vegetable Patties
calories 507; KJ 2117; protein 23g; fat 2g; saturated fat 13g; fibre 4g; sodium 575mg; calcium 500mg

p.173 Spiced Tofu Burgers
calories 160; KJ 669; protein 8g; fat 9g; saturated fat 1g; fibre 2g; sodium 85mg; calcium 322mg

p.174 Roasted Thai-style Tofu with Stir-fried Vegetables
calories 290; KJ 1208; protein 15g; fat 17g; saturated fat 2g; fibre 5g; sodium 986mg; calcium 681mg

p.176 Marinated Tofu with Satay Sauce
calories 452; KJ 1877; protein 19g; fat 36g; saturated fat 7g; fibre 3g; sodium 772mg; calcium 348mg

p.177 Hot Spiced Chickpeas
calories 175; KJ 741; protein 9g; fat 5g; saturated fat 0.6g; fibre 6g; sodium 264mg; calcium 64mg

p.177 Chickpea & Potato Stew
calories 393; KJ 1654; protein 17g; fat 12g; saturated fat 1g; fibre 10g; sodium 693mg; calcium 149mg

p.178 Mixed Beans with a Cornmeal Topping
calories 544; KJ 2290; protein 30g; fat 18g; saturated fat 8g; fibre 13g; sodium 1955mg; calcium 438mg

p.179 Butternut Squash & Gruyère Risotto
calories 537; KJ 2230; protein 17g; fat 30g; saturated fat 13g; fibre 3g; sodium 399mg; calcium 373mg

p.181 Roasted Vegetable Lasagne
calories 473; KJ 1986; protein 25g; fat 23g; saturated fat 11g; fibre 5g; sodium 423mg; calcium 505mg

p.181 Pappardelle with Spicy Tomato Sauce & Ricotta
calories 392; KJ 1659; protein 15g; fat 10g; saturated fat 4g; fibre 4g; sodium 149mg; calcium 177mg

p.182 Broccoli & Gruyère Souffle
calories 245; KJ 1016; protein 13g; fat 18g; saturated fat 10g; fibre 1g; sodium 259mg; calcium 286mg

p.183 Mediterranean Stuffed Peppers with Coucous
calories 434; KJ 1802; protein 14g; fat 26g; saturated fat 7g; fibre 3.2g; sodium 864mg; calcium 160mg

p.186 French Beans with Feta & Sun-dried Tomatoes
calories 125; KJ 511; protein 4g; fat 10g; saturated fat 3g; fibre 1g; sodium 400mg; calcium 95mg

p.186 Roasted Baby Carrots with Feta & Sun-dried Tomatoes
calories 160; KJ 670; protein 6g; fat 10g; saturated fat 15g; fibre 3g; sodium 202mg; calcium 188mg

p.187 Asian-style Broccoli
calories 75; KJ 310; protein 5g; fat 5g; saturated fat 1g; fibre 3g; sodium 224mg; calcium 72mg

p.188 Honeyed Parsnips with Sesame Seeds
calories 250; KJ 1069; protein 4g; fat 14g; saturated fat 7g; fibre 8g; sodium 113mg; calcium 125mg

p.189 Fantail Roast Potatoes with Sesame Seeds
calories 304; KJ 1218; protein 7g; fat 9g; saturated fat 1g; fibre 4g; sodium 22mg; calcium 50mg

p.190 Sweet Potato & Anchovy Gratin
calories 650; KJ 2707; protein 14g; fat 50g; saturated fat 29g; fibre 4g; sodium 610mg; calcium 321mg

p.190 Aubergine & Tomato Gratin
calories 334; KJ 1384; protein 9g; fat 31g; saturated fat16g; fibre 2g; sodium 273mg; calcium 186mg

**p.192 Cauliflower & Broccoli Cheese**
calories 520; KJ 2167;
protein 13g; fat 48g;
saturated fat 29g; fibre 3g;
sodium 457mg;
calcium 296mg

**p.192 Apple, Walnut & Watercress Salad**
calories 223; KJ 936; protein 3g;
fat 20g; saturated fat 2g;
fibre 2g; sodium 15mg;
calcium 63mg

**p.193 Potato Salad with Blue Cheese Dressing**
calories 250; KJ 1039;
protein 11g; fat 13g;
saturated fat 8g; fibre 2g;
sodium 311mg;
calcium 136mg

**p.196 Fudgy Nut Pie**
calories 615; KJ 2580;
protein 8g; fat 32g;
saturated fat 12g; fibre 2g;
sodium 470mg;
calcium 75mg

**p.196 Spiced Apple & Raisin Pancakes**
calories 338; KJ 1434;
protein 8g; fat 5g;
saturated fat 1.5g; fibre 4g;
sodium 172mg;
calcium 155mg

**p.197 Rich Chocolate & Fig Puddings with Chocolate Sauce**
calories 6240; KJ 2612;
protein 10g; fat 33g;
saturated fat 19g; fibre 2g;
sodium 477mg;
calcium 156mg

**p.198 Dates Stuffed with Ricotta**
calories 180; KJ 766; protein 4g;
fat 5g; saturated fat 2g;
fibre 1.5g; sodium 53mg;
calcium 82mg

**p.198 Brandied Prunes with Crème Fraîche**
calories 149; KJ 629; protein 3g;
fat 3g; saturated fat 2g; fibre 2g;
sodium 33mg;
calcium 67mg

**p.199 Lemon & Strawberry Cheesecake**
calories 800–600; KJ 3342–2507;
protein 8–6g; fat 57–43g;
saturated fat 34–26g;
fibre 2–1.5g;
sodium 560–419mg;
calcium 206–154mg

**p.201 Caramel Oranges with Almond & Sesame Seed Biscuits**
calories 455; KJ 1921;
protein 6g; fat 14g;
saturated fat 5g; fibre 3g;
sodium 92mg;
calcium 123mg

**p.202 Mixed Berry Brulée**
calories 240; KJ 1011;
protein 6g; fat 7g;
saturated fat 4g; fibre 1.5g;
sodium 62mg;
calcium 130mg

**p.202 Lemon & Passion Fruit Roulade**
calories 350; KJ 1465;
protein 6g; fat 15g;
saturated fat 8g; fibre 1g;
sodium 84mg;
calcium 80mg

**p.203 Apricot Risotto**
calories 480; KJ 1996;
protein 14g; fat 17g;
saturated fat 8g; fibre 3g;
sodium 175mg;
calcium 353mg

**p.204 Frozen Strawberry Yogurt**
calories 241; KJ 1008;
protein 9g; fat 11.5g;
saturated fat 6g; fibre 1g;
sodium 100mg;
calcium 210mg

**p.204 Lemon Mascarpone Ice Cream**
calories 490; KJ 2037;
protein 4g; fat 42g;
saturated fat 25g;
fibre 0g; sodium 258mg;
calcium 94mg

**p.208 Sun-dried Tomato & Parmesan Corn Bread Squares**
calories 200; KJ 830;
protein 7g; fat 10g;
saturated fat 4g; fibre 0.5g;
sodium 504mg;
calcium 130mg

**p.208 Cheese & Watercress Scones**
calories 240; KJ 1025;
protein 8g; fat 11g;
saturated fat 7g; fibre 1g;
sodium 375mg;
calcium 329mg

**p.209 Parmesan & Herb Twists**
calories 80; KJ 330; protein 1g;
fat 5g; saturated fat 0.5g;
fibre 0g; sodium 73mg;
calcium 24mg

**p.210 Soda Bread**
(per slice) calories 174; KJ 741;
protein 7g; fat 2g; saturated fat
0g; fibre 4g; sodium 493mg;
calcium 64mg

**p.210 Banana & Pumpkin Loaf**
(per slice) calories 240; KJ 1004;
protein 4g; fat 9g;
saturated fat 1g; fibre 2g;
sodium 137mg;
calcium 77mg

**p.211 Sesame Oat Crisps**
calories 100; KJ 415; protein 1g;
fat 6g; saturated fat 2g;
fibre 0.5g; sodium 95mg;
calcium 22mg

**p.213 Almond & Pine Nut Cookies**
calories 111; KJ 462; protein 2g;
fat 7g; saturated fat 3g;
fibre 0.5g; sodium 64mg;
calcium 22mg

**p.214 Apricot & Orange Muffins**
calories 245; KJ 1031;
protein 5g; fat 9g;
saturated fat 5g; fibre 1g;
sodium 365mg;
calcium 90mg

**p.214 Citrus Yogurt Cake**
calories 565; KJ 2365;
protein 9g; fat 31g;
saturated fat 18g;
fibre 1.5g; sodium 266mg;
calcium 156mg

**p.215 Lemon & Poppy Seed Drizzle Loaf Cake**
calories 335; KJ 1399;
protein 6g; fat 19g;
saturated fat 11g; fibre 3g;
sodium 254mg;
calcium 94mg

**p.216 Rich Chocolate Cake**
calories 520; KJ 2155;
protein 8g; fat 36g;
saturated fat 16g;
fibre 1.5g; sodium 193mg;
calcium 80mg

**p.216 Carrot Cake with Mascarpone Topping**
calories 747; KJ 3103;
protein 10g; fat 60g;
saturated fat 29g;
fibre 2g; sodium 427mg;
calcium 131mg

# Index

## Exercise index

Ankle 26, 42
Arm 36, 64, 66
Aquaerobics 83

Back 16, 36, 44–9
Balance 10, 21, 26, 36, 38–43, 83, 93
BMD (bone mineral density) 5, 6, 93
  age-related loss 7
  and exercise 7, 13, 21, 36–7
Body weight 13
Bone-loading 6, 13, 21
Bone development 7
  DXA scan 8
  structure 5, 6
  turnover 6
Brittle bones see osteoporosis

Calcium 6, 12
  absorption problems 9
  adequate intake (AI) 12
  sources of 12
Calf 30–31
Cardiovascular problems 93
Chest 32, 70
Circulation exercises 22–3, 24
Clothing 18, 88, 91
Contraceptive pill 9

Dancing 90
Diet 12
Dowager's hump 10
Drugs 11

Eating disorders 9
Equipment 20
Ethnic group 9
Exercise, benefits of 4, 5, 6, 7, 11, 21
  choosing the right kind 13
  getting the most from 19
  personal programme 20, 94–5

Falls 38, 93
Family history 8, 9
Fractures see osteoporotic fracture

Gender 8
Gut conditions 9
Gym 37, 54, 70, 86–7

Health 92, 93
Hip 10, 11, 48, 50, 52, 54, 56, 58, 60, 84, 88, 91
HRT (hormone replacement therapy) 8, 9, 11, 88
Hysterectomy 8

Jogging 54, 91
Joints 22
Jumping 54, 88–9

Kidney conditions 9

Leg 36, 48–61
Lifting 16

Menopause 5, 7, 8, 11, 12
  early menopause 8
  pre- & post- 12, 21, 37, 60, 72, 90
Mobility exercises 22–3, 26–7, 28–9
Muscles 22–3, 24
  adaptability 30

Oestrogen 7, 8, 9, 11
Osteoarthritis 78, 91, 93
Osteoporosis 4–11, 93
Osteoporotic fracture 5, 6, 7, 9, 10, 13, 21, 62
  weak spots 10

Pelvic floor muscles 17
Pelvic tilt 14–15
Posture 14–15, 16, 21, 30

Reflexes 22
Running 91

Shoes 88, 91
Shoulder 26–7, 68–9
  flexibility 46–7
  frozen shoulder 46
Smoking 10
Spine 10, 14, 15, 28–9, 32–3, 48, 60, 70, 84, 91
Stair climbing 82
Steroid treatment 9
Stretching 21, 22–3, 30–35, 78–9
Studio classes 90
Synovial fluid 28

T'ai Chi Ch'uan 83
Thigh 30–31, 52–3, 60–61
Thyroid problems 9

Vitamin D 12

Walking 24–5, 81
  barefoot 30–31
  walk–jog 81, 84–5
Warning signs 19
Weight-training 20, 37, 80, 86–7
Wrist 10, 62–3, 66, 68, 70, 72, 74–5

## Recipe index

Entries in italics denote variations on the main recipes

Almond & Pine Nut
  Cookies 213
Apple
  Apple, Walnut & Watercress
    Salad 192
  & Blueberry Muesli 106
  Spiced Apple & Raisin
    Pancakes 196
Apricot
  & Orange Muffins 214
  & Orange Smoothie 109
  Risotto 203
Asian-style Broccoli 187
Aubergine & Tomato Gratin 191
Avocado & Smoked Salmon
  Rolls 123

Bacon & Ricotta Tart 138
Bagels with Raspberries &
  Ricotta 108
Baked Ricotta with Roasted Vine
  Tomatoes 120
Banana
  & Almond Smoothie 108
  & Pumpkin Loaf 210
Beef
  Blue Cheese & Walnut
    Steaks 156
  Meatballs with Mozzarella &
    Tomato Sauce 157
  Minced Beef with Polenta
    Topping 159
  *Minced Beef with Olive & Stilton
    Polenta Topping 159*
Biscuits
  Almond & Pine Nut
    Cookies 213
  Caramel Oranges with
    Almond & Sesame Seed
    Biscuits 201
  Sesame Oat Crisps 211
Blue Cheese
  Potato Salad with Blue Cheese
    Dressing 193
  *Soufflés 135*
  & Walnut Steaks 156
Brandied Prunes with Greek
  Yogurt 198
Breads
  Banana & Pumpkin Loaf 210
  Soda Bread 210
  Sun-dried Tomato & Parmesan
    Corn Bread Squares 208
Brie-stuffed Chicken with
  Creamy Pesto 142
Broccoli
  Asian-style Broccoli 187

Cauliflower & Broccoli
  Cheese 192
Cod & Broccoli Cheese Pie 163
  & Gruyère Soufflé 182
  *Salmon & Broccoli Cheese Pie
    163*
  & Smoked Ham Tagliatelle 151
  & Stilton Soup 116
Butternut Squash & Gruyère
  Risotto 179

*Caesar Salad on Toasted Ciabatta
  133*
Cajun Cheese Potato Skins with
  Tomato & Red Onion
  Salad 136
Cakes
  Carrot Cake
    with Mascarpone
    Topping 216
    *with Orange Mascarpone
    Topping 217*
  Citrus Yogurt Cake 214
  Lemon & Poppy Seed Drizzle
    Loaf Cake 215
  Rich Chocolate Cake 216
Caramel Oranges with Almond
  & Sesame Seed Biscuits 201
Carrot Cake
  with Mascarpone
    Topping 216
    *with Orange Mascarpone
    Topping 217*
Cauliflower & Broccoli Cheese
  192
Cheese & Leek Sausages 172
Cheese & Watercress Scones 208
Cheesy Scrambled Eggs 111
Cherry Tomato & Goat's Cheese
  Tartlets 122
Chicken
  Brie-stuffed Chicken with
    Creamy Pesto 142
  Caesar Salad with Parmesan
    Crisps 133
  Coronation Chicken Salad 144
  Garlic Chicken in Yogurt 143
  & Sesame Bites 145
  Tikka Salad 132
  & Wild Mushroom
    Stroganoff 143
Chickpea
  Hot Spiced Chickpeas 177
  Moroccan Spiced Chickpea
    Soup 116
  & Potato Stew 177
  *& Sweet Potato Stew 177*
Chocolate
  Fudgy Nut Pie 196
  Rich Chocolate Cake 216
  Rich Chocolate & Fig
    Puddings with Chocolate
    Sauce 197

Citrus Yogurt Cake 214
Cod
 & Broccoli Cheese Pie 163
  *with Carrot Topping* 163
  *with Parsnip Topping* 163
 Baked in Yogurt 164
Coronation Chicken Salad 144
Creamy Guacamole 124
Croque Monsieur 130

Dates Stuffed with Ricotta 198
Deep-fried Whitebait 165
Dips
 Creamy Guacamole 124
 Humous 128
 Red Pepper Humous 128
 Roasted Red Pepper Dip 124
 Tzatziki 124
Dried Fruit Spread 108

Egg(s)
 Cheesy Scrambled Eggs 111
 Feta Omelette with Rocket &
  Red Pepper 134
 Smoked Haddock Omelette
  111
 Soft Eggs with Soured Cream
  & Smoked Salmon 112

Falafel with Salad in Pitta 129
Fantail Roast Potatoes with
 Sesame Seeds 189
Feta Omelette with Rocket & Red
 Pepper 134
Fish (*see also* individual fish)
 Deep-fried Whitebait 165
 Griddled Swordfish with Salsa
  Verde 167
 Monkfish Kebabs with
  Roasted Vegetables and
  Pesto 166
 Penne with Prawns &
  Asparagus 168
 Pie with Rosti Topping 165
 Prawn & Spinach Roulade 168
 *Tuna Kedgeree* 162
French Beans with Feta &
 Sun-dried Tomatoes 186
French Onion Soup 119
*Fresh Pesto* 142
Frozen Strawberry Yogurt 204
Fruit (*see also* individual fruit)
 Brandied Prunes with Greek
  Yogurt 198
 Caramel Oranges with
  Almond & Sesame Seed
  Biscuits 201
 Dates Stuffed with Ricotta 198
 Dried Fruit Spread 108
 Mixed Berry Brulée 202
 Spiced Fruit Compote 107
Fudgy Nut Pie 196

Garden Pea & Watercress Soup
 with Sesame Croutons 119
Garlic & Cumin Roasted Lamb
 with Apricot & Chickpea
 Salsa 153
Garlic Chicken in Yogurt 143

Griddled Swordfish with Salsa
 Verde 167
*Grilled Vegetables with Satay
 Sauce* 176

Haddock
 Poached Haddock with
  Spinach & Poached Egg 164
 Smoked Haddock &
  Sweetcorn Chowder 120
 Smoked Haddock &
  Sweetcorn Fritters 113
 Smoked Haddock Omelette
  111
*Home-made Caesar Salad
 Dressing* 133
Honeyed Parsnips with Sesame
 Seeds 188
Hot Spiced Chickpeas 177
Humous 128

Ices
 Frozen Strawberry
  Yogurt 204
 Lemon Mascarpone Ice
  Cream 204

Lamb
 Garlic & Cumin Roasted Lamb
  with Apricot & Chickpea
  Salsa 153
 *Moroccan Lamb with Butter
  Beans & Prunes* 154
 Moroccan Lamb with
  Chickpeas & Apricots 154
 Moussaka 155
 Shepherd's Pie 156
 Skewered Lamb with Tomato,
  Chilli & Yogurt Marinade
  152
Lemon
 & Passion Fruit Roulade 202
 & Poppy Seed Drizzle Loaf
  Cake 215
 *& Raspberry Cheesecake* 199
 & Strawberry Cheesecake 199
 Mascarpone Ice Cream 204

Marinated Tofu with Satay
 Sauce 176
Meatballs with Mozzarella &
 Tomato Sauce 157
Mediterranean Stuffed Peppers
 with Couscous 183
Mixed Beans with a Cornmeal
 Topping 178
Mixed Berry Brulée 202
Monkfish Kebabs with Roasted
 Vegetables & Pesto 166
Moroccan Lamb with Chickpeas
 & Apricots 154
*Moroccan Lamb with Butter Beans
 & Prunes* 154
Moroccan Spiced Chickpea
 Soup 116
Moussaka 155
*Mushroom Polenta* 150
Mushrooms & Goat's Cheese in
 Aubergine Parcels 121

Pappardelle with Spicy Tomato
 Sauce & Ricotta 181
Parmesan & Herb Twists 209
*Parsnips with a Sweet Lime
 Glaze* 188
Pasta
 Broccoli & Smoked Ham
  Tagliatelle 151
 Pappardelle with Spicy
  Tomato Sauce & Ricotta 181
 Penne with Prawns &
  Asparagus 168
 Pork with Pak Choi & Black
  Bean Sauce 148
 *Vegetable Tagliatelle* 151
Pastry
 Cherry Tomato & Goat's
  Cheese Tartlets 122
 Fudgy Nut Pie 196
 Parmesan & Herb Twists 209
 *Pesto & Parmesan Twists* 209
 Smoked Salmon & Dill
  Quiche 161
 Spiced Spinach, Lentil & Feta
  Filo Pie 171
Penne with Prawns &
 Asparagus 168
Peppered Smoked Mackerel
 Spread 132
*Pesto & Parmesan Twists* 209
Poached Haddock with Spinach
 & Poached Egg 164
Polenta with Bacon &
 Mushrooms 150
Pork
 Escalopes with Celeriac Cream
  Mash 148
 Stuffed with Apricots & Pine
  Nuts 146
 *Stuffed with Apple &
  Walnuts* 146
 with Pak Choi & Black Bean
  Sauce 148
Potato(es)
 Cajun Cheese Potato Skins
  with Tomato & Red Onion
  Salad 136
 Fantail Roast Potatoes with
  Sesame Seeds 189
 Fish Pie with Rosti
  Topping 165
 *Red Pesto Fantail Roast
  Potatoes* 189
 Salad with Blue Cheese
  Dressing 193
 Spinach & Potato Cake 139
 Sweet Potato & Anchovy
  Gratin 190
 Sweet Potato with Cottage
  Cheese & Crispy Bacon 139
Prawn & Spinach Roulade 168

Quick Ciabatta Pizza 130
Quick Salmon Kedgeree 162
Quick Turkey Cassoulet 145

Red Pepper Humous 128
*Red Pesto Fantail Roast Potatoes*
 189

Rice
 Apricot Risotto 203
 Butternut Squash & Gruyère
  Risotto 179
 Quick Salmon Kedgeree 162
 *Tuna Kedgeree* 162
Rich Chocolate & Fig Puddings
 with Chocolate Sauce 197
Rich Chocolate Cake 216
Roasted Baby Carrots with
 Parmesan & Coriander
 Topping 188
Roasted Pepper Soup with Feta &
 Basil 117
Roasted Red Pepper Dip 124
Roasted Thai-style Tofu with
 Stir-fried Vegetables 174
Roasted Vegetable Lasagne 181

Salads
 Apple, Walnut & Watercress
  Salad 192
 *Caesar Salad on Toasted
  Ciabatta* 133
 Cajun Cheese Potato Skins
  with Tomato & Red Onion
  Salad 136
 Coronation Chicken Salad 50
 Potato Salad with Blue Cheese
  Dressing 193
 Tomato & Mozzarella Salad
  122
 Warm Lentil & Feta Salad 170
 Watercress, Pear & Roquefort
  Salad 123
Salmon
 Avocado & Smoked Salmon
  Rolls 123
 *& Broccoli Cheese Pie* 163
 Fish Cakes 160
 *& Leek Lasagne* 160
 Quick Salmon Kedgeree 162
 Smoked Salmon & Dill
  Quiche 161
 with a Crumb Crust 162
Sesame Oat Crisps 211
Shepherd's Pie 156
Skewered Lamb with Tomato,
 Chilli & Yogurt Marinade
 152
Smoked Salmon & Dill Quiche
 161
Smoothies
 Banana & Almond 108
 Apricot & Orange 109
 Strawberry 109
Soda Bread 210
Soft Eggs with Soured Cream &
 Smoked Salmon 112
Soufflés
 Blue Cheese 135
 Broccoli & Gruyère 182
 *Spinach & Gruyère* 182
 Twice-baked Goat's Cheese 134
Soups
 French Onion Soup 119
 Garden Pea & Watercress Soup
  with Sesame Croutons 119

Moroccan Spiced Chickpea Soup 116
Roasted Pepper Soup with Feta & Basil 117
Spiced Apple & Raisin Pancakes 196
Spiced Fruit Compote 107
Spiced Spinach, Lentil & Feta Filo Pie 171
Spiced Tofu Burgers 173
Spicy Roasted Baby Carrots with Feta 186
Spinach
  & Gruyère Soufflé 182
  Poached Haddock with Spinach & Poached Egg 164
  & Potato Cake 139
  Prawn & Spinach Roulade 168
  & Roquefort Pancakes 136
  Spiced Spinach, Lentil & Feta Filo Pie 171
Strawberry Smoothie 109

Stuffed Portobello Mushrooms 113
Sun-dried Tomato & Parmesan Corn Bread Squares 208
Sweet Fruit Porridge 106
Sweet Potato & Anchovy Gratin 190
Sweet Potato with Cottage Cheese & Crispy Bacon 139

Tofu
  Marinated Tofu with Satay Sauce 176
  Roasted Thai-style Tofu with Stir-fried Vegetables 174
  Spiced Tofu Burgers 173
Tomato(es)
  Aubergine & Tomato Gratin 190
  Baked Ricotta with Roasted Vine Tomatoes 120
  Cherry Tomato & Goat's

Cheese Tartlets 122
  & Mozzarella Salad 122
Tuna Kedgeree 162
Twice-baked Goat's Cheese Soufflés 134
Tzatziki 124

Vegetable(s) (see also individual vegetables)
  Cauliflower & Broccoli Cheese 192
  French Beans with Feta & Sun-dried Tomatoes 186
  Grilled Vegetables with Satay Sauce 176
  Honeyed Parsnips with Sesame Seeds 188
  Mediterranean Stuffed Peppers with Couscous 183
  Mushroom Polenta 150
  Mushrooms & Goat's Cheese in Aubergine Parcels 121

Parsnips with a Sweet Lime Glaze 188
Patties 172
Roasted Baby Carrots with Parmesan & Coriander Topping 92
Roasted Vegetable Lasagne 87
Spicy Roasted Baby Carrots with Feta 186
Stuffed Portobello Mushrooms 113
Tagliatelle 151

Warm Lentil & Feta Salad 170
Watercress, Pear & Roquefort Salad 123
Welsh Rarebit 130

## Useful addresses

**National Osteoporosis Society** Manor Farm, Skinners Hill, Camerton, Bath, BA2 0PJ, (01761) 471771, www.nos.org.uk

**Physical Company** Cherry Cottage, Hedson Rd, Bourne End, Bucks, (01628) 520208

**Forza Fitness Equipment Ltd** 58–60 St Katherine's Way, London, E1W 1LR, (020) 7816 5300, kate.Wilde@forzagroup.com

**UK T'ai Chi Association** PO Box 159, Bromley, Kent, BR1 3XX, (020) 8289 5166

## References

■ E. Bassey, M. Rothwell et al. *Pre- and postmenopausal women have different bone mineral density responses to the same high-impact exercise.* J Bone Miner Res 1998; 13:1805–13.

■ C. Coupland, S. Cliffe et al. *Habitual physical activity and bone mineral density in postmenopausal women in England.* Int J Epidemiol 1999; 28:241–6.

■ D. Kerr, A. Morton et al. *Exercise effects on bone mass are site-specific and load dependent.* J Bone Miner Res 1996; 11:218–25.

■ W. Kohrt, D. Snead et al. *Additive effects of weight-bearing exercise and estrogen on bone mineral density in older women.* J Bone Miner Res 1995; 10:1303–11.

■ E. A. Krall, B. Dawson-Hughes. *Walking is related to bone density and rates of bone loss.* Am J Med 1994; 96:20–6.

■ T. Lohman, S. Going et al. *Effects of resistance training on regional and total bone mineral density in premenopausal women: A randomized prospective study.* J Bone Miner Res 1995; 10:1015–24.

■ M. Revel, M. Mayou-Benhamou et al. *One-year psoas training can prevent lumbar bone loss in postmenopausal women: a randomised controlled trial.* Calcif Tissue Int 1993; 53:307–11.

■ M. Sinaki, B. A. Mikkelsen. *Postmenopausal spinal osteoporosis: flexion versus extension exercises.* Arch Phys Med Rehabil 1984; 65:593–6.

■ C. Snow-Harter, M. L. Bouxsein et al. *Effects of resistance and endurance exercise on BM status of young women: a randomized exercise intervention trial.* J Bone Miner Res 1992; 7:761–9.

■ L. Welsh, O. M. Rutherford. *Hip bone mineral density is improved by high-impact aerobic exercise in postmenopausal women and men over 50 years.* Eur J Appl Physiol 1996; 74:511–7.

The publishers would like to thank the authors for their help in combining *Great Healthy Food for Strong Bones* and *Exercise for Strong Bones.*

Picture Credits from *Exercise for Strong Bones*
8 (bottom) Prof. P. Motta/Dept of Anatomy/University 'La Sapienza', Rome/SPL, 56 Getty Images Stone, 62 Getty Images Stone, 64 Thomas Hart Shelby/Retna, 85 Telegraph Colour Library, 89 Getty Images Stone